A Practical Guide to Female Sexual Medicine

The appropriate diagnosis, management, and even terminology for women with sexual health problems have all been much debated in the past few years. This practical text aims to guide the gynecologists, urologists, family physicians, and other professionals involved with the care of these patients. With case presentations, treatment algorithms, and schematic illustrations, this comprehensive yet accessible text will be an invaluable reference for the current state of the clinical art.

A Practical Guide to Female Sexual Medicine

Corey R Babb, DO, FACOOG, IF, MSCP

Medical Director
The Haven Center for Sexual Medicine &
Vulvovaginal Disorders
Tulsa, Oklahoma

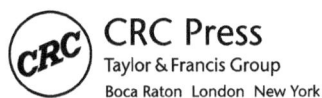

CRC Press
Taylor & Francis Group
Boca Raton London New York

CRC Press is an imprint of the
Taylor & Francis Group, an **informa** business

Designed cover image: Getty Images

First edition published 2025
by CRC Press
2385 NW Executive Center Drive, Suite 320, Boca Raton, FL 33431

and by CRC Press
4 Park Square, Milton Park, Abingdon, Oxon, OX14 4RN

CRC Press is an imprint of Taylor & Francis Group, LLC

ISBN: 978-1-032-79924-7 (hbk)
ISBN: 978-1-032-77121-2 (pbk)
ISBN: 978-1-003-49452-2 (ebk)

DOI: 10.1201/9781003494522

Typeset in Minion
by Apex CoVantage, LLC

Contents

SECTION I   Core Concepts in the Practice of Female Sexual Medicine

SECTION II   Domains of Female Sexual Dysfunction

SECTION III   Evaluation and Management of the Female Sexual Medicine Patient

Preface

The purpose of this guide is to provide the practitioner with a handbook to help navigate the ever-changing and complex world of female sexual medicine. It is not intended to be the "end all, be all" sexual medicine textbook, as to try and create such a document in the (relatively) new discipline of female sexual medicine would be a sign of hubris and nearsightedness. Instead, I hope that the chapters contained within provide a blueprint to help the provider navigate the treatment of these often-complex patients. When possible, I have included a flow chart to allow for some idea of treatment regulation, but understand that no sexual medicine patient is alike – their individual histories and concerns keep the "standardized" patient from being a reality – and as such, feel free to deviate from the chart if situations warrant.

To help facilitate learning, and to also provide a quick reference, I have organized the book into three sections. Section I, "Core Concepts in the Practice of Female Sexual Medicine," introduces the foundational principles in sexual medicine, focusing on patient autonomy, the nuances of addressing sensitive topics in clinical settings, and the anatomical and physiological facets of female sexual function. It aims to prepare clinicians with a strong baseline understanding of both the biological and psychological aspects of sexual function. Section II, "Domains of Female Sexual Dysfunction," dives into the specific domains of sexual dysfunction – desire, arousal, pain, and orgasm. Each chapter covers function and dysfunction in these areas and provides an in-depth exploration of the conditions associated with each domain, as well as a discussion on pathophysiology and specific "buzzwords" that may help the practitioner ask pertinent questions for diagnosis. Finally, Section III, "Evaluation and Management of the Female Sexual Medicine Patient," focuses on the diagnosis and treatment of female sexual disorders, covering diagnostic tests, therapeutic interventions, and lifestyle factors. It provides clinicians tools for comprehensive assessment and management, including pharmacologic, surgical, and nonmedical treatment modalities. Each chapter concludes with a case study, so that the provider can see how the information in the chapter may be used in a real-life situation.

Above all, I hope that this guide allows the clinician to feel comfortable treating female sexual medicine patients – at least at a basic level. With the staggering amount of sexual dysfunction present, it is a travesty that so many patients feel alone in their treatment journey. That said, most patients would like their providers to ask the initial questions about sexual wellness, so I implore you to take that first step and ask – you never know what response you may get!

Acknowledgments

No book is born in isolation, and neither is an author alone in its creation. My deepest gratitude goes out to those who walked with me on this journey, whose guidance, love, and support shaped the words on these pages.

First and foremost, to God be the glory – without His grace, none of this would be possible.

To my editor, Robert Peden, thank you for your belief in this vision and for granting me the opportunity to share this knowledge with others.

To my patients, who inspire me daily with their resilience and trust and remind me why this work matters.

To my parents, Ray and Jannelle, whose unwavering love and steadfast encouragement taught me the value of perseverance and the importance of always seeing things through.

To my mentors and colleagues – Peter Pacik, Nisha McKenzie, Sally MacPhedran, Aleece Fosnight (whose wisdom shaped the section on sexual minority patients), Heather Howard, and Melanie Modjoros – your insights, support, and experiences have been invaluable in formulating the content of these pages.

To Kimberly Magana, my dedicated beta reader and research companion, thank you for your tireless optimism and for helping access sources from the OSUMC library!

And finally, to my incredible wife, Emily – you are ever my muse. Your faith in me, your patience, and your boundless love made this book possible.

Author

Dr. Corey R Babb is a board-certified gynecologist; a Fellow of the International Society for the Study of Women's Sexual Health (ISSWSH), where he serves on the board of directors; a Menopause Society Certified Menopause Practitioner (MSCP); a member of the International Society for the Study of Vulvovaginal Disorders (ISSVD); and a reviewer for multiple sexual medicine journals.

Section I

Core Concepts in the Practice of Female Sexual Medicine

Chapter 1

The Female Sexual Medicine Patient

At the time of this writing, there are approximately 3.95 billion women on planet Earth.[1] Of those women, approximately 50% of them are currently struggling with some form of sexual dysfunction.[2] To put that figure into perspective, approximately 1.9 billion women – more than the population of India – have sexual dysfunction. That number is staggering. Despite this fact, the sexual concerns of female patients are some of the least discussed, least taught, and least treated facets of modern medicine. From an objective standpoint, this makes no sense. We know that the act of sexual intercourse is undoubtedly the most important action taken for the continuation of the species and that, artificial reproduction aside, the female participant is half of that equation. Why, then, is women's sexual health not given more consideration in medical training?

Much of this disconnect can be attributed to the schism between sex for conception and sex for recreation. Sex for conception is necessary, and therefore it is "OK," at least from a cultural standpoint. For women who have difficulty with conception, an entire branch of medicine – reproductive endocrinology and infertility – exists, and if need be, the act of sex can be removed from conception entirely. For women who have difficulty with sex for recreation, however, the story is less straightforward. Concerns about low sexual desire are often placated with statements such as "It's because you're a mom" or "You're too stressed." Painful intercourse? "Drink some wine, it will relax you" or "You're just too tight. Have

DOI: 10.1201/9781003494522-1

more sex to loosen things up." Patients who are unable to orgasm are told "That's OK, a lot of women don't orgasm." Imagine a patient who presents with a broken wrist being told to "break your wrist more, it will help." This is exactly the type of recommendation many patients with sexual medicine concerns receive, however, and to put it bluntly, such advice is neither scientifically valid nor supportive of patient care.

In this chapter, we will discuss the initial facets to the evaluation of the female sexual medicine patient. The concepts of patient autonomy and informed consent will be reviewed, as well as specific topics related to trauma-informed care, privacy, and navigating sensitive issues. Finally, the Standardized Sexual Medicine Exam, a focused way to evaluate patients with sexual concerns, will also be explained. These topics will be integrated into further chapters and help build the foundation for the practice of female sexual medicine.

1.1 Patient Autonomy and Informed Consent

To better understand how medical professionals can address these disparities, it is critical to explore foundational principles such as autonomy and informed consent. First discussed by the philosophers Immanuel Kant and John Stuart Mill, the concept of personal autonomy evolved from the idea that "persons have intrinsic and unconditional worth, and therefore, should have the power to make rational decisions and moral choices."[3] When extrapolated to healthcare, this ideal is retitled as patient autonomy and is considered one of the cornerstones of medical ethics. In short, patient autonomy governs the patient's ability to make decisions about their body, as well as their medical care. For patients with sexual concerns, the ability to assert this autonomy is paramount when addressing deeply personal and intimate aspects of their history. Recognizing and respecting patient autonomy involves fostering an environment where patient voices are heard, preferences acknowledged, and decisions honored. For the sexual medicine provider, giving patients agency to actively participate in their treatment and medical decision making not only cultivates trust in the patient-provider relationship but also fosters a sense of ownership of their sexual health.

Similarly, the concept of informed consent serves as an ethical gatekeeper for upholding standards in healthcare delivery, *especially* as it pertains to sexual dysfunction. Informed consent entails providing the patient with comprehensive information regarding their condition and treatment options, as well as associated risks, benefits, and alternatives for those therapies. For patients presenting with sexual concerns, the discussion of treatment choices can be fraught with emotion, especially if they have been the victim of medical gaslighting for their symptoms. As such, the sexual medicine provider should provide a candid yet compassionate discourse, ensuring that patients are equipped with the knowledge and understanding necessary to make the most appropriate decision regarding their care. Much like autonomy, discussing the use of appropriate diagnostic and therapeutic tools in a way that allows for informed consent adds to the relationship between the patient and their provider and helps ensure that the patient retains agency over their own healthcare. In summary, recognizing and respecting patient autonomy and ensuring informed consent are cornerstones of building trust and creating effective treatment strategies in female sexual medicine. As we move into the discussion of trauma-informed care and standardized exams, these ethical principles will continue to underpin our approach to addressing the sexual health needs of women

1.2 Navigating Sensitive Topics and Privacy Concerns

Despite the high prevalence of female sexual dysfunction, the subject remains almost taboo in modern society. As such, discussing sexual concerns, even in the medical setting, often requires mixing both a delicate approach to the discourse and the use of compassionate language from the healthcare provider. Additionally, it behooves the sexual medicine provider to remember that every patient faces a unique bias towards sexual issues. Cultural stigmas, religious beliefs, or even current relationship factors may bring about feelings of guilt or shame when discussing sexual concerns. It is therefore essential to establish a safe and nonjudgmental environment where patients feel comfortable expressing their concerns, with providers employing empathetic communication skills, including active listening, validation of concerns, and nonjudgemental discussion. To facilitate this, providers may want to employ the SOLER[4] (**S**it squarely; **O**pen posture; **L**ean towards the other; **E**ye contact; **R**elax) technique during patient history taking.

Just as cultural, religious, and relationship dynamics shape a patient's views on sexual health, past trauma can also have profound effects on their sexual wellbeing. Unfortunately, upwards of 60% of patients may have experienced a form of sexual or genital trauma in the past,[5] and roughly 70% of those patients relate their sexual issues to that trauma.[6] Providers should therefore use trauma-informed care (TIC) during the evaluation of the sexual medicine patient. According to the Substance Abuse and Mental Health Services Administration, TIC "realizes the widespread impact of trauma and understands potential paths for healing; recognizes the signs and symptoms of trauma in staff, clients, and others involved with the system; and responds by fully integrating knowledge about trauma into policies, procedures, practices, and settings."[7] For the sexual medicine provider, using the AACE (Acknowledge, Agency, Consent, Education)[8] guide to the

TABLE 1.1 AACE Guide

Acknowledge	Acknowledge that the patient has different pelvic experiences than the provider.
Agency	The patient is in charge of their body. Allow them to guide the exam.
Consent	Ask for consent to examine prior to the exam.
Education	Discuss the reason for the exam, as well as findings acquired during the exam.

trauma-informed pelvic exam may allow patients to feel more in charge of their care and ultimately remove or reduce the amount of trauma that invasive examinations can produce (Table 1.1).

Finally, patients may express or harbor fears about their personal health information (PHI) being disclosed without consent. As sexual concerns are innately very personal, this concern is logical. Therefore, in addition to standard privacy practices, healthcare providers should maintain strict confidentiality standards, ensuring that discussions about sexual health issues with other providers, family members, etc., remain confidential unless explicitly authorized by the patient. As such, it is recommended that any transmission of PHI to other healthcare providers be preceded by a patient-signed specific release of information form (an example is provided in Appendix 2) listing the specific healthcare information to be transmitted. If preferred, some providers may elect to give a physical copy of the patient's records at the conclusion of the visit, so that the patient can ultimately decide who has access to their PHI. Finally, offering private consultation spaces and guaranteeing discretion during appointments can be reassuring to the patient, ultimately establishing the rapport needed to help navigate sexual concerns without fear of judgment or breach of confidentiality.

BOX 1.1   SEXUAL MINORITY PATIENTS

It is well documented that individuals who identify as a sexual minority face unique barriers to medical care.[9] As such, clinicians may also consider the following practices to ensure that patients feel welcomed and valued, regardless of gender or sexual orientation:

1. *Include inclusive language with all patients.* The use of appropriate pronouns, sexual orientation terms, and person-first language not only creates an inclusive space for patients to express their concerns but also brings attention to the diversity present in the sexual medicine clinic regardless of sexual orientation and identity.
2. *Understand barriers to care for sexual minorities.* Many individuals who identify as a sexual minority face, or have faced, significant healthcare discrimination in the form of fear, stigma,

or embarrassment by previous providers. Understanding and acknowledging these concerns may help strengthen the patient-provider relationship and allow patients to feel more at ease discussing their concerns

3. *Patients who practice alternative sexual practices*, such as bondage/domination/sadomasochism (BDSM), kink, or polyamory, may be uncomfortable discussing specific concerns related to their sexual lifestyle. Providers should therefore educate themselves about these and other sexual practices and be comfortable using appropriate terminology when discussing them with patients. Additionally, reassuring patients that their concerns will be addressed regardless of sexual practice may allow them to be more open when discussing sensitive topics.

4. *Provide inclusive sexual health education for all patients, including those who identify as a sexual minority*. Sexual minority groups, especially sexual and gender minority youths, demonstrate higher rates of sexually transmitted infections as well as unintended pregnancies.[10] It is therefore essential that the sexual medicine provider take the necessary time to ask about safe sex practices, consensual sexual activities, and, if appropriate, contraceptive options in addition to overall sexual wellbeing.

1.3 The Standardized Sexual Medicine Examination

While the standard pelvic exam provides a basic evaluation of the female genital tract, the Standardized Sexual Medicine Examination (SSME) allows for a more thorough examination of the genital structures that may lead, or contribute to, sexual concerns as well as a way to document or record pertinent findings that can aid in diagnosis (Table 1.2). The following section reviews the components of the SSME, as well as the tools needed to perform the evaluation; Chapter 2 provides in-depth information on the specific anatomic structures.

1.3.1 Performing the SSME

When performing the SSME, providers may wish to follow this protocol to allow for both ease of charting and to assure that they do not accidentally miss any of the structures noted in the table. An examination template may be found in Appendix 3.

After obtaining appropriate consent, the patient is placed in a relaxed, semi-Fowler's position. First, a visual inspection of the groin and vulva is performed, with any anomalies noted. Attention is paid to the hair follicles,

TABLE 1.2 The Standard Sexual Medicine Examination Quick Chart

Anatomic Location	Specific Structures	Possible Findings (Not Exhaustive)
Groin	Inguinal crease	Excoriations Erythematous plaques Stellate papules/pustules Ulcerations
Vulva	Mons pubis	Excoriations Pigment changes Lesions Pubic hair changes Pigmented lesions
	Labia majora and infralabial sulci	Thickening Atrophy Pigment changes Masses/nodules Tenderness Erythema Vesicles Pigmented lesions
	Labia minora	Atrophy Retraction Erythema Vesicles Pigmented lesions
	Clitoris	Tenderness Loss of sensation Phimosis Adhesions Keratin pearls Pigment changes Pigmented lesions
	Posterior commissure	Excoriations Tenderness Fissures Pigment changes Scarring Pigmented lesions
Vestibule	Anterior vestibule	Erythema Tenderness Hyperemia Papilloma Milia Cystic masses
	Urethra	Caruncle Papilloma Erythema Tenderness
	Skene's glands	Erythema Tenderness

TABLE 1.2 *(Continued)* The Standard Sexual Medicine Examination Quick Chart

Anatomic Location	Specific Structures	Possible Findings (Not Exhaustive)
	Posterior vestibule	Erythema Tenderness Hyperemia Papilloma Milia Cystic masses Fissuring
	Posterior fourchette	Erythema Tenderness Fissuring
	Bartholin glands	Enlargement Cystic mass Tenderness
Vagina	Anterior vaginal wall	Prolapse Absent or varying rugae Tenderness Mass
	Posterior vaginal wall	Prolapse Absent or varying rugae Tenderness Mass
	Apex	Prolapse Granulation tissue Mass Pigmented lesions
Pelvic floor	Pubococcygeus	High tone Low tone Tenderness Spasm
	Iliococcygeus	High tone Low tone Tenderness Spasm
	Obturator internus	High tone Low tone Tenderness Spasm
	Puborectalis	High tone Low tone Tenderness Spasm
	Voluntary contraction (Kegel)	Absent contraction Tetany with relaxation
Anus		Excoriations Fissuring Color change Erythema

as well as any changes in the skin, including atrophic thinning or lichenification. The labial structures, including the infralabial sulcus, are then palpated for any masses or nodules, and if applicable, neurogenital testing (discussed in Chapter 8) may be performed. The clitoral hood is then gently retracted, and the glans clitoris is examined for obvious pathology. If a clitoral phimosis is present, the degree should be documented. Additionally, it is important to evaluate the tissue underneath the clitoral hood for any accumulations of debris, smegma, or hardened collections of squamous cells, coined "keratin pearls." If present, the location and number of clitoral adhesions should be reported as well. The perineum is then evaluated for fissuring, skin changes, or other lesions, and the overall caliber of the perineal body should be documented as well. Finally, evaluation of the perianal tissue should occur, with attention paid to changes in pigment, as well as any fissures or excoriations.

Second, the labia minora are then gently separated and the vestibule is evaluated for visual changes, beginning at the anterior aspect of the vestibule and progressing posteriorly. Of note, documentation of abnormal findings along the vestibule is usually described in "clockface" fashion (2 o'clock, 4 o'clock, etc.). A cotton-tip applicator is then used to gently palpate the vestibule to assess for any degree of tenderness or discomfort. The same applicator may be used to also evaluate the urethra and periurethral tissues and evaluate for discomfort. The Skene's glands, located in the 1 and 11 o'clock position of the vestibule, should be assessed for tenderness and inflammation of their ostia. Attention is then turned to the bilateral Bartholin glands, which should be palpated for inflammation or pain. Finally, the posterior fourchette should be examined for excoriations, fissures, or erythema.

For the vaginal portion of the SSME, the author recommends a small, plastic speculum for the majority of patients. While there are many techniques that allow for relatively trauma-free insertion of the device, the author has found that once the tip of the speculum is on the introitus, firm, digital pressure along the groin, roughly in the area of Alcock's canal, can be used as a distraction technique to minimize insertional discomfort. Once inserted, the speculum may then be opened to assess for internal pathology and then rotated 90 degrees to allow for visualization of the urethral bulb, as well as anterior and posterior vaginal walls. When removing the speculum, the author has found that timing the removal of the device with exhalation may provide reduction in discomfort.

Finally, to evaluate the pelvic floor, the author recommends using the index finger on the provider's dominant hand. With insertion of the finger, the initial tone of the vaginal introitus should be noted, and if pain is present, the provider should attempt to have the patient report where the pain is most localized. If possible, the finger should then be inserted past the hymenal ring and a lateral curling motion utilized to assess the muscles of the pelvic floor. Providers should note the tone of the muscle (high or low) and whether the palpation produces a painful sensation. Palpation of the pelvic floor may also elicit other sensations from the patient, such as the urge to void or defecate, and this should be recorded as well. If applicable, the sacrospinous ligaments may be palpated at roughly the 4 and 8 o'clock position, and pain documented. Finally, voluntary contraction of the introital muscles should be elicited, and the strength of the response, as well as additional recruitment of abdominal or gluteal muscles, noted.

1.3.2 Tools and Techniques

Two tools are paramount to performing the SSME: vulvoscopy and adequate lighting. While many healthcare providers are familiar with colposcopy as a means to evaluate the cervix and vagina, the word vulvoscopy may be unfamiliar. Simply put, vulvoscopy is the visual inspection of the vulva and vestibule, utilizing a device that allows for additional magnification of the genitalia. The standard colposcope may be used for vulvoscopy, and the technique for placement and setup is the same. Additionally, should the evaluator feel that there is a need to visualize the vagina, a speculum can be inserted and the vulvoscope "converted" to a colposcope (Figure 1.1). In terms of lighting, a vulvoscope can provide the appropriate amount

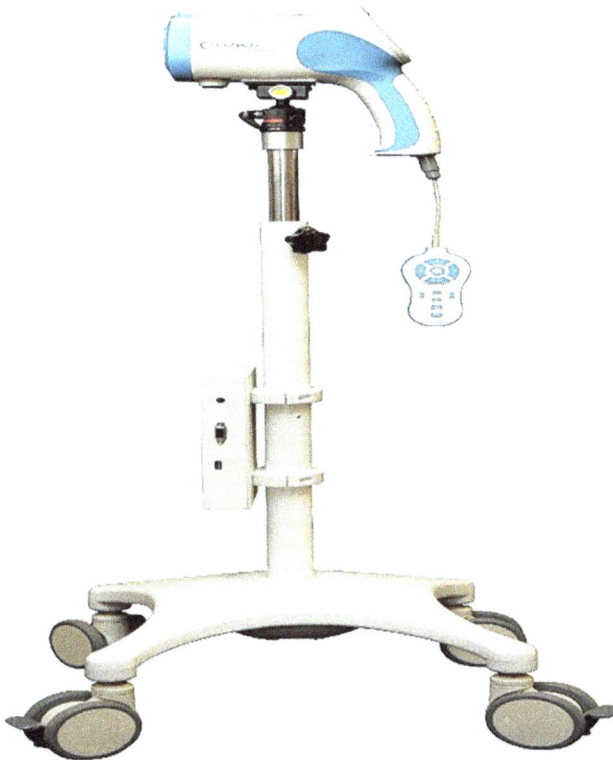

FIGURE 1.1   Colposcope. (Courtesy of Lutech Medical.)

of lighting needed, but should that be unavailable, the practitioner may use a headlamp, a stand lamp, or have an assistant hold a lighting device. Regardless of the method utilized, the importance of good lighting cannot be understated.

1.4 Conclusion

The core concepts in the evaluation of the female sexual medicine patient are intrinsically no different from that performed on a non–sexual medicine patient. Patient autonomy, informed consent, and trauma-aware practices should be the norm in any modern medical setting. Even the SSME is simply a more specialized evaluation of a specific body system and similar in thoroughness to the type of examination an ophthalmologist would give to a patient's eye or a podiatrist to their feet. What makes the evaluation of the sexual medicine patient unique is that many patients with sexual concerns have poor understanding of their own anatomy[11] and therefore may have a difficult time properly describing where their concerns, at least anatomically, lie. It is up to the provider therefore to allow patients to feel comfortable in explaining their symptoms and discuss their concerns in a completely nonjudgmental way. By helping patients feel a sense of agency in their healthcare decisions and making sure that they understand the facets of their care, the sexual medicine provider can be a champion in preventing medical trauma to the patient.

1.5 Case Study

Harriet is a 17-year-old female, G0, who presents to the clinic for evaluation of a painful "spot on my vagina." She states that she noticed the lesion approximately one week ago and that the area itched for approximately 48 hours prior to becoming apparent. Her mother brings her to the office and is currently sitting in the exam room with her. You sense that the patient may not be telling the whole truth but is anxious with her mother present. You do have a chaperone present in the exam room. Which of the following is not an effective way of establishing rapport with this patient?

  A: Discussing patient confidentiality as part of the evaluation and how her HPI is protected

  B: Asking that, with the patient's permission, her mother leave the exam room so that you can ask personal questions and explaining that you do this with all teenage patients

  C: Leaving the exam room door open to the hallway during your discussion

  D: Using the SOLER method during your discussion

The answer is C. Assuring the patient that your conversation will be confidential and that her PHI is protected may help assuage her fears. In addition, as long as you have a chaperone present, asking other family members to step out of the room so that you can ask questions about sexual history or other, more personal concerns can be helpful in relieving patient anxiety. Leaving the exam room door open does not provide the private space that many patients want to discuss sexual concerns. The SOLER method is an effective way to improve rapport with patients.

Chapter 2

Female Sexual Anatomy

2.1 External and Internal Genital Anatomy

Sexual anatomy is separated into two main divisions: external and internal. While both facets of anatomy are important for sexual function, one cannot simply lump them together in terms of discussion. Despite being colloquial labeled as "the vagina," the difference between said vagina and the vulva, for instance, is immense. In addition to the basic architecture, one must also be familiar with manifestations of the nervous system, as well as the divisions of the pelvic floor in each specific section, as multiple pathologies derive from aberrancies in those areas.

Historically, the term "vagina" did not exist in medical textbooks until the 1700s, and in antiquity it was believed that the female pelvic organs "wandered around the abdomen," causing illness when they crashed into other internal organs such as the liver or pancreas. Despite myriad changes in the practice of medicine and the understanding of the body since the ancient Greeks, the vagina and vulva – and their contained structures – have remained mostly undisturbed in our collective understanding. It has only been recently that we have mapped and understood the nerves of the clitoris, for example, and while that should be celebrated, one must not forget that there are literally thousands of healthcare practitioners that routinely call the vulva the vagina and are not

DOI: 10.1201/9781003494522-2

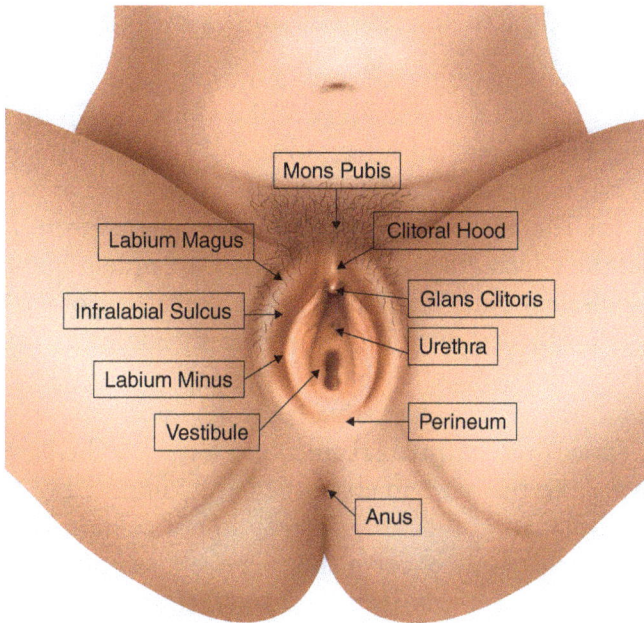

FIGURE 2.1   The external genitalia.

aware of their inaccuracy. If one were to, for instance, call the nose the face, many a raised eyebrow would occur. Not so for the female genitalia.

Regardless, the sexual medicine practitioner must be aware of the specific anatomic structures of the vulva, vagina, and associated structures, and care should be taken to not only use their correct name but also to educate the patient on what is "normal" in terms of appearance, coloration, etc. (Figure 2.1). It is only by enlightening the public to these specifications that we can move the science of sexual anatomy into the 21st century.

2.1.1 The Vulva

The term "vulva" etymologically arises from the Latin word *volva*, which translates loosely to "womb." There may also be some derivation from the verb *volere*, meaning "to twist" or "to wrap." As it stands, the vulva has three noticeable landmarks: the mons pubis, the labia (separated into the external labia majora and internal labia minora), and the clitoris. The vulva receives its arterial blood supply from the pudendal arteries, venous drainage from the internal pudendal vein, lymphatic effluence to the inguinal lymph nodes, and nervous input from branches of the pudendal nerve, perineal nerve, and ilioinguinal nerve. The vulva has a significant number of estrogenic receptors, and physical changes in appearance are noticeable at puberty, pregnancy, and after menopause.

Specific details of the structures in Figure 2.2 are as follows:

Mons pubis: The mons pubis is a fat pad overlying the pubic symphysis that forms the superior boundary of the vulva. It provides padding during penetrative sexual intercourse and also contains numerous hair follicles from which pubic hair originates.

Labia majora: The labia majora (*sing.* labium magus) form the lateral border of the vulva. They are composed of squamous epithelial cells, but have distinct outer and inner layers, consisting of darker, more keratinized skin, with hair follicles on the outside, and a thinner, less keratinized layer ripe with sebaceous glands.

Labia minora: The labia minora (*sing.* labium minus) are separated from the labia majora by infralabial sulci and form the medial border of the vulva. Like the labia majora, they are composed of squamous epithelial cells but, unlike the majora, do not contain hair follicles. They merge superiorly to form the prepuce, or hood of the clitoris, and terminate posteriorly in the posterior fourchette of the introitus. The labia minora often have the greatest degree of variation in the external genitalia and are the main structure associated with the cosmetic labioplasty procedure.

Clitoris: The clitoris is a protrusion of the embryologic genital tubercle and is considered the primary female sexual organ. It does not have a purpose other than pleasure and is estimated to house 10,000 nerve endings or more.[12] The clitoris is divided into three main structures: the glans, the body (made up of the erectile corpora cavernosa), and

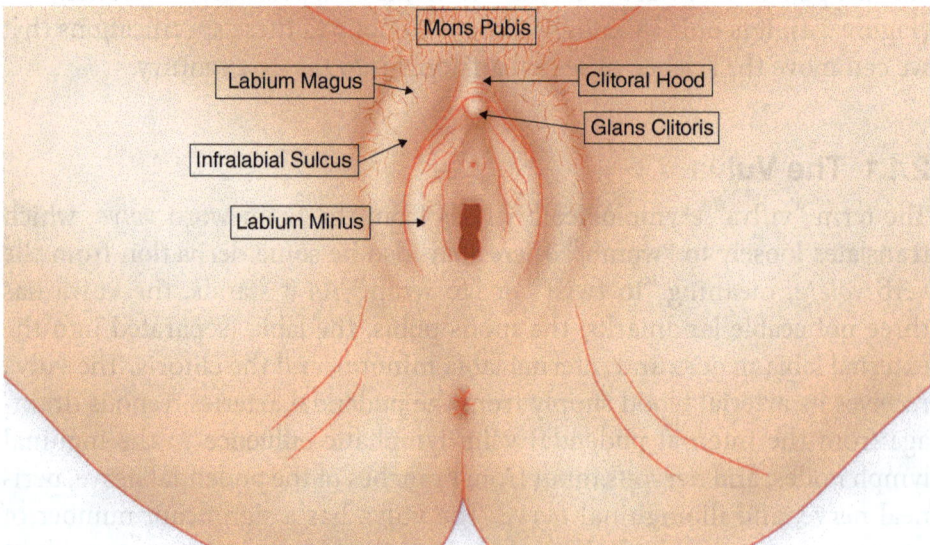

FIGURE 2.2   The vulva.

the crura, or legs, that wrap around the vaginal introitus. With sexual arousal, the clitoris will become erect, swelling with blood from the earlier-mentioned vasculature. In addition, the clitoris is rich in hormone receptors for both estrogens and androgens. The main nervous input for the clitoris comes from the superior branch of the pudendal nerve, although there is significant innervation from the dorsal nerve of the clitoris as well.

2.1.2 The Vestibule

The vestibule, also known as the vulval vestibule, vulvar vestibule, or vestibule of the vagina, is technically considered part of the vulva but has enough unique characteristics to be discussed on its own. Anatomically, it exists between the labia minora and the vagina and is demarcated by Hart's line externally and the hymenal ring internally. It is an area rich in androgen receptors, as it is embryologically derived from the urogenital sinus, an area with a significant amount of both estrogen and testosterone activity. Of note, the vestibule does not contain significant amounts of keratinized epithelium, making it significantly more sensitive to chemical additives or allergens when compared to the vulva. Other important structures within the vestibule include the Bartholin glands, the Skene glands, and the distal portion of the urethra. As mentioned earlier, the hymen is also part of the vestibule and may be found intact or separated when performing a vulvar exam. The vestibule also contains the entrance to the vagina, known as the introitus. See Figure 2.3.

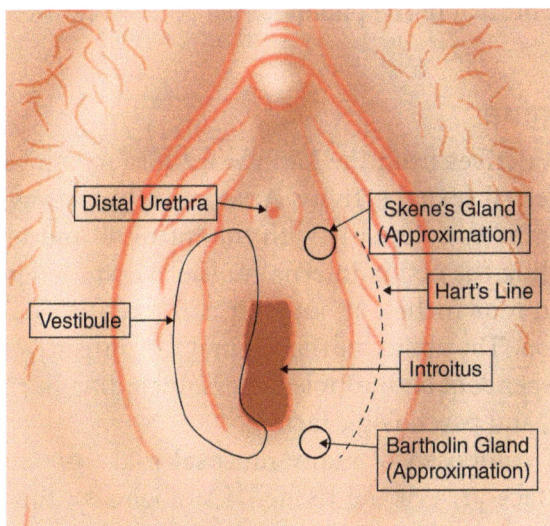

FIGURE 2.3   Vestibule.

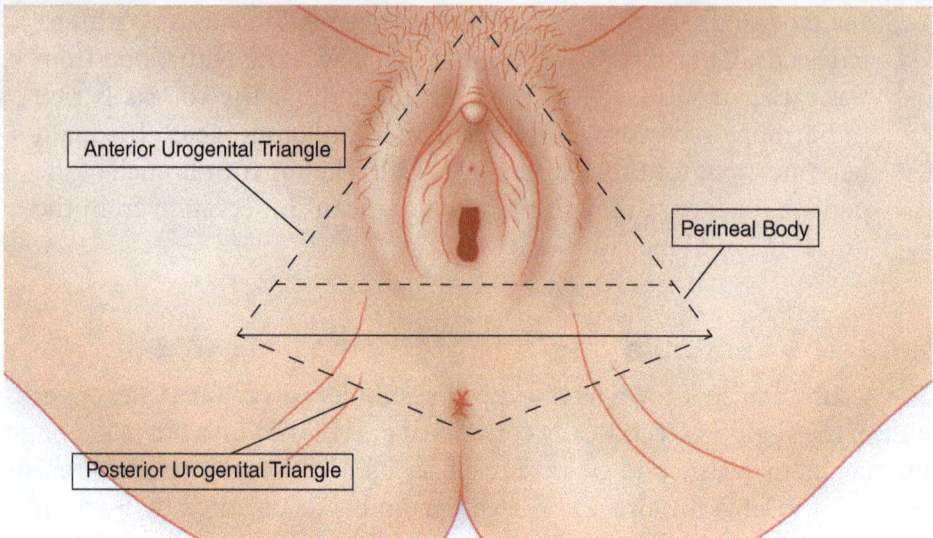

FIGURE 2.4   Perineum.

2.1.3 The Perineum

The perineum is the total surface space between the pubic symphysis and the coccyx. Anatomically, it is divided into two separate "urogenital triangles," bordered laterally by the ischial tuberosities, with apexes at the pubic arch anteriorly and the coccyx posteriorly. The anterior urogenital triangle houses the external genitalia, and the posterior urogenital triangle contains the anus. The transverse perineal muscle acts as a border between the triangles and helps contribute to the perineal body. Blood flow to the perineum comes from the perineal artery, while the main sensory nerve input comes from the middle branch of the pudendal nerve. See Figure 2.4.

2.1.4 The Vagina

The term vagina derives from the Latin word for "sheath" and is the main structure for internal sexual activity. Anatomically, the vagina is a muscular tube that originates externally with the introitus and terminates at the fornix, surrounding the cervix internally. The average length of a vagina is between two and four inches, although it can roughly double in size with sexual stimulation. The ability of the vaginal introitus to stretch and allow penetration is dependent on multiple factors, including hormonal presence, pelvic floor tone, and psychologic factors.

The vagina is composed of many mucosal folds, or "rugae," that help increase the surface area of the tissue. Histologically, the vagina is composed of superficial and intermediate cells, as well as an underlying parabasal cell layer. The superficial cells are both fluid filled and rich in glycogen

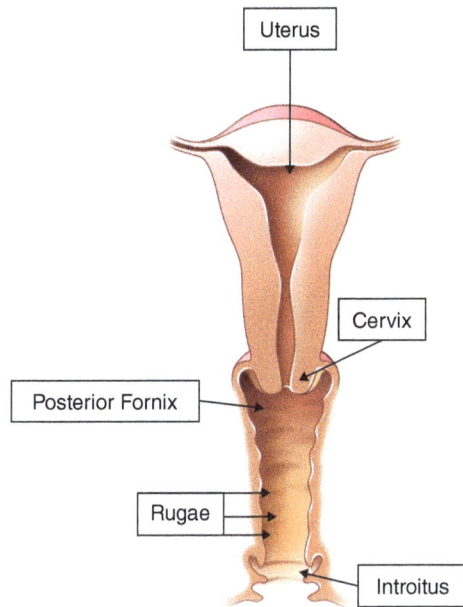

FIGURE 2.5 The vagina.

and are incredibly resistant to tearing and trauma. It is the abundance of these superficial cells that allows for the vagina to stretch with vaginal deliveries. Comparatively, the parabasal cells act as a scaffolding for the vaginal tissue and are not well suited to accommodate stretch or trauma.

The vascular flow to the vagina is mainly from the vaginal artery, although both the uterine artery and the internal pudendal artery provide circulatory input as well. Venous drainage occurs from the uterovaginal venous plexus and the vaginal vein. The main nerves to the vagina include innervations from the pelvic plexus superiorly and the pudendal nerve inferiorly. See Figure 2.5.

2.1.5 The Pelvic Floor

Arguably the most important muscular structure for sexual activity, the pelvic floor, also (incorrectly, as they are two separate entities) known as the pelvic diaphragm, is a group of muscles that separate the pelvic cavity from the perineal tissue. It is composed of the coccygeus (also known as the ischiococcygeus) and levator ani muscle, as well as associated fascia and connective tissue. The levator ani muscle group is specifically composed of three muscles: the pubococcygeus, the iliococcygeus, and the puborectalis.

The function of the pelvic floor is myriad, including holding the pelvic viscera in place, aiding with urination and defecation, maintaining posture, and ambulation. Sexually, it contracts with orgasm, and spasm in any or all

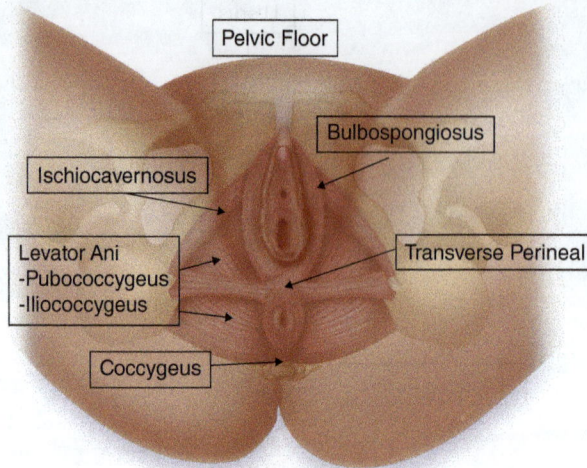

FIGURE 2.6 **The pelvic floor.**

the muscles noted earlier can lead to pain with penetration, or even complete inability to tolerate sexual activity. Defects or weakening in the pelvic floor are referred to as prolapses and are further delineated by their location and severity.

Vascular arterial flow to the pelvic floor occurs via the inferior gluteal, inferior vesical, and pudendal arteries. Venous drainage occurs via the internal, external, and common iliac veins and their associated tributaries. Innervation occurs mainly from the lumbosacral trunk (L4–S3), as well as sacral and coccygeal plexuses. See Figure 2.6.

2.1.6 The Anus

The anus represents the terminal end of the digestive tract and serves as an exit to allow passage of stool from the intestinal tract, via a process known as defecation. Despite having a primary function that is not sexual in nature, anal stimulation is a common component of sexual activity for people of all sexual orientations and therefore should not be ignored. Anatomically, the anus is separated from the genitalia by the perineum and located inside the intergluteal cleft. It contains two muscular rings, called sphincters, that control the passage of stool and gas.

Arterial flow to the anus comes from the middle and inferior rectal arteries, and venous drainage occurs from similarly named veins. Innervation to the anus is mainly from the pudendal nerve. Sexual stimulation of the anus in female patients occurs mostly from indirect stimulation to the vagina and crura of the clitoris, although stretching of the anal sphincters alone may elicit a pleasurable sensation to some individuals.

2.1.7 Conclusion

While an understanding of female sexual anatomy is helpful for any practitioner, it is even more important for the sexual medicine provider. As noted earlier, each structure plays a unique role in the orchestration of the female sexual experience, while maintaining necessary bodily function for digestion, parturition, and, in the case of the pelvic floor, activities of daily living. It is simply not feasible to ignore sexual anatomy and expect to deliver quality care. Additionally, the sexual medicine provider should be a champion of normalization – that is to say, changing public opinion that these terms, especially genital ones, are "dirty words." Correct delineation of the vulva, vestibule, and vagina will help with this as well, as hopefully society can move beyond lumping these very different parts into one colloquial term for female genital anatomy.

2.2 Sexual Response Cycle

The idea of a separate physiology for sexual activity is not a new one, with erotic texts describing sexual arousal and orgasm existing as early as 400 BCE with the classical Indian text, *Kama Sutra*, which mentions even older Vedic prose about sexuality. In the 20th century, Alfred Kinsey published two works, *Sexual Behavior in the Human Male* and *Sexual Behavior in the Human Female* in 1948 and 1953, respectively, which paved the way for societal "acceptance" of human sexuality, but it was not until Masters and Johnson published their landmark *Human Sexual Response* in 1966 that the idea of a medically accurate human sexual physiology gained scientific approval (Figure 2.7). Since that publishing, multiple other sexual response models

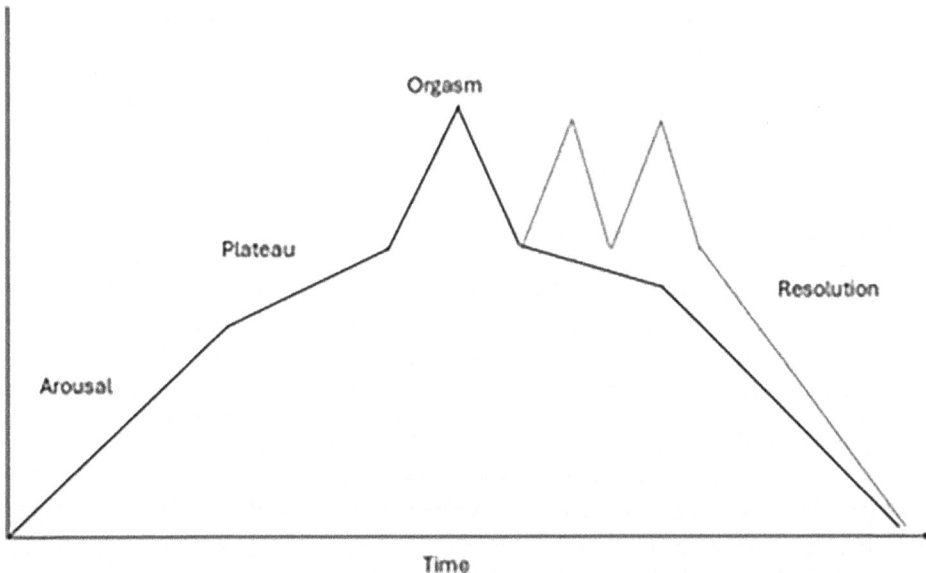

FIGURE 2.7   The Masters and Johnson sexual response model.

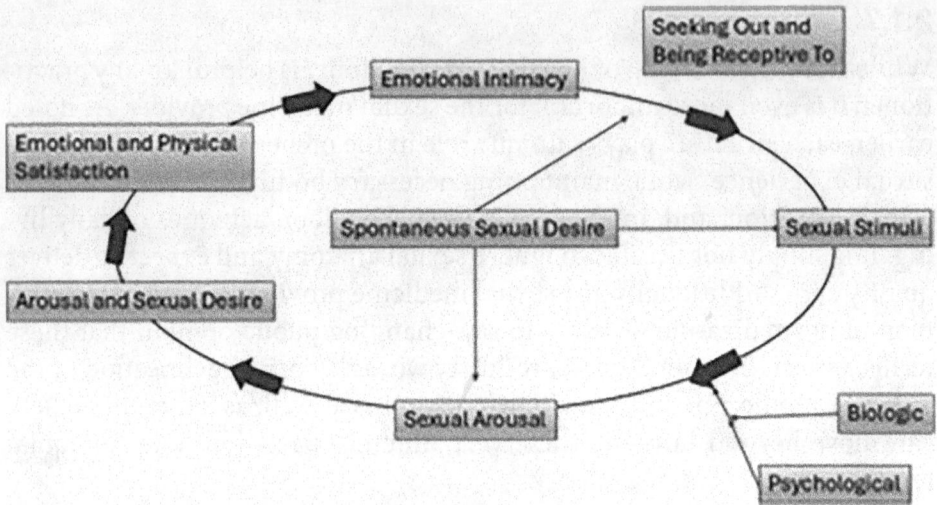

FIGURE 2.8 The Basson sexual response model.

have been formulated, with Rosemary Basson's circular model (Figure 2.8) considered the most accurate in terms of a specific female sexual response.

As one can see, the Basson model appears to be realistic in that, unlike the Masters and Johnson model which stipulates a resting "excitement phase," the individual begins from a sexually neutral position and only after certain criteria are met do they advance towards desiring sexual activity. Regardless, one cannot deny that the Masters and Johnson model does have its merits in that it fully delineates separate stages of sexual physiology, which will be explained in detail later.

The author is aware that there are multiple criticisms of the Masters and Johnson model but has decided to use it to help explain different components of sexual physiology at a basic level. The author notes that this model does not consider variances in psychological, behavioral, or relationship status.

2.2.1 Excitement Phase

Physiologically speaking, the excitement phase is synonymous with sexual arousal, which is the physical and psychological manifestation of desire. Arousal is mediated by the parasympathetic nervous system (PNS), which causes blood to flow to the genitals via preganglionic innervation from the sacral spinal cord, as well as somatic motor innervation from α-motor neurons in the ventral horn of lower spinal cord segments.[13] Nerve impulses from S2–S4 sacral segments lead to activation of the postganglionic neurons, which allow for vasodilation to occur in the reproductive organs. In addition, a cascade of reproductive and adrenal hormones, namely testosterone, prolactin, estrogens, and, to a lesser extent, cortisol, cause vasocongestion of the skin (flushing), nipple erection, engorgement of the vulva, and lubrication of the vagina.

2.2.2 Plateau Phase

The plateau phase is accompanied by an increase in heart rate and respiration. The same PNS activity is present during this phase, although it is intensified, and for patients who are unable to achieve orgasm, this phase can often be the peak of their sexual experience. Further changes in the genitalia are present, including narrowing of the introitus via tightening of the pubococcygeus muscle, widening of the vaginal sidewalls, production of further secretions from the Bartholin glands, and increased sensitivity in the clitoris.

2.2.3 Orgasm Phase

The orgasm phase represents the shift in autonomic control from the PNS to the sympathetic nervous system (SNS). It is controlled via preganglionic sympathetic innervation from the thoracic and lumbar spinal segments, specifically T11–L2, which causes vasoconstriction, shunting blood away from the genitalia. This switch in autonomic control leads to a reflex from the previously mentioned spinal cord α-motor neurons, causing involuntary muscle contractions of the pelvic floor. In some individuals, these contractions may also be accompanied by uncontrolled vocalizations, eye movements, or spasming accessory muscles in the extremities. Of note, the cervix will "dip" into the vaginal fornix with orgasm to ease the passage of semen into the uterus.

2.2.4 Resolution Phase

As blood continues to leave the genitalia, heart rate and respirations return to a preexcitatory level, called the resolution phase. Blood pressure also drops during this time, which may contribute to the "postcoital headache" encountered by some individuals. The duration of the resolution phase is variable and may last from minutes to hours, especially in older individuals. In addition, Masters and Johnson reported a "refractory period" during the resolution phase during which further orgasm was impossible in men, although women were able to achieve repeat orgasms if significant stimulation occurred.[14] This idea is contested, however, as there are accounts of women having similar refractory periods in the literature.[15]

2.2.5 Conclusion

Female sexual physiology is a complex dance that cannot simply be distilled into graphs or diagrams. While the components of the physiologic process may be straightforward to discuss, the specific process behind them is highly individual. One cannot simply apply the previous methods, whatever they may be, to every situation. Autonomic innervation cannot be controlled, and its activity should not be an indication of the thought processes behind the sexual response. There exists an incredibly erroneous thought that unwanted arousal or orgasm is a subconscious manifestation of sexual desire. This cannot be further from the truth. A rape victim having an orgasm during that experience does not mean that "they wanted it," and a person who suffers with persistent genital arousal disorder becoming aroused during a car ride does not mean that they are hypersexual. Our bodies respond to impulses/signals from nerves whether we want them to or not. It is the thought behind that response that truly gives it sexual significance.

2.3 Sexual Endocrinology

A thorough understanding of sexual endocrinology is important for the sexual medicine practitioner. Historically, humans have been using hormonal extracts as early as 200 BCE, with Chinese texts describing the process of isolating gonadal hormones for medicinal purposes from human urine. In 1849, Arnold Berthold first described the effects of testicular hormones on capons (castrated roosters) after noticing a return of secondary sexual characteristics such as aggression, crowing, and wattle growth when rooster testicles were transplanted into the capons' abdomens. It was not until the 1930s, however, that manufactured testosterone was available for medicinal use. In terms of estrogens, similar animal experiments were performed, and, once again, the 1930s saw the development of synthesized estrogen compounds. Likewise for progesterone.

*Before delving into endocrine specifics, it is important to note the naming structure of the hormone. The suffix -gen signifies the family that the hormone is derived from. For example, estradiol is a type of estro**gen**, testosterone is a type of andro**gen**, and so forth. To use the term estrogen to describe the effects of estradiol is incorrect. Also, the suffix -tin implies that the hormone is synthetic, as in a proges**tin** versus a naturally occurring progesterone, which is, in itself, a progestogen.*

When discussing disorders that involve gonadal hormones, it is important to understand their effects on the body. As such, we will begin with the most important premenopausal hormonal cycle for sexuality: the menstrual cycle (Figure 2.9).

The menstrual cycle occurs over the course of approximately 28 days. The cycle is divided into two halves, which are dependent on whether ovulation has occurred. In a 28-day cycle, ovulation will occur on approximately

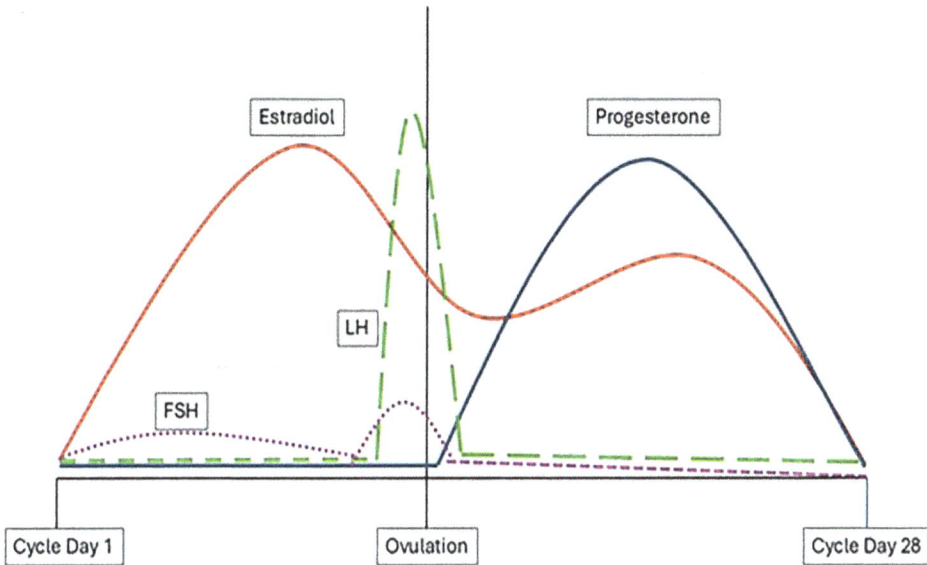

FIGURE 2.9   The menstrual cycle.

day 14. The portion of the cycle that occurs prior to ovulation is termed the follicular phase, with the portion that follows ovulation termed the luteal phase. The first day of menses is noted as cycle day 1. When discussing the endometrium, the terms "follicular" and "luteal" are replaced with "proliferative" and "secretory," respectively. The duration of the follicular phase may vary due to a variety of factors. Conversely, the luteal phase is dependent on the lifespan of the corpus luteum, which requires human chorionic gonadotropin (HCG) to survive. As such, individuals with longer or shorter menstrual cycles are in fact demonstrating the varying length of the follicular phase – the length of the luteal phase is mostly static at an average of 14 days.

BOX 2.1

The menstrual cycle is an expression of a mature hypothalamic–pituitary–ovarian (HPO) axis, the hormonal highway that controls gonadal hormone production. The HPO axis (Figure 2.10) is an example of a negative feedback system, where elevated levels of "downstream" hormones cause cessation of their respective stimulating hormones "upstream." Obviously, the converse is true as well, as lower levels of "downstream" hormones elicit a release of "upstream" stimulating hormone.

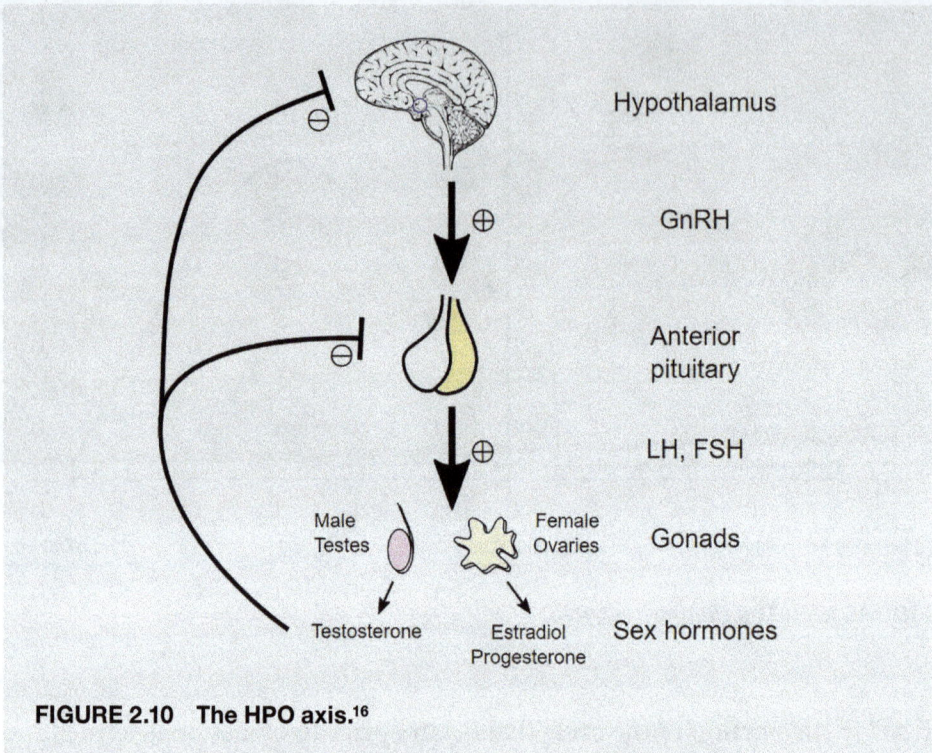

FIGURE 2.10 The HPO axis.[16]

2.3.1 Follicular Phase

The sexually mature hypothalamus produces gonadotropin-releasing hormone (GnRH) in a pulsatile fashion, which travels to the anterior pituitary via the hypophyseal portal system. Once there, it binds to receptors on the pituitary, causing the release of follicle-stimulating hormone (FSH) and luteinizing hormone (LH) into the bloodstream. These two hormones are called gonadotropins. Once FSH reaches the ovary, it reacts with ovarian granulosa cells to stimulate follicular growth, eventually leading to the formation of a solitary dominant follicle. LH acts on the dominant follicle, causing it to release even more estradiol via production of androstenedione, an estrogen and androgen prohormone, until the follicle fully matures.

2.3.2 Ovulation

Once maturation is complete, a release of 17α-hydroxyprogesterone from the dominant follicle temporarily inhibits estradiol release, while at the same time stimulating a massive "LH surge" from the pituitary, which lasts approximately 24 to 48 hours. This surge in LH triggers ovulation, as well as initiates the development of the corpus luteum from the previous dominant follicle. Once ovulated, the human egg will "live" for approximately 12 to 24 hours before dissolving, typically in the fallopian tube, unless fertilization occurs. Contrary to popular belief, missing an ovary will not cause one to only ovulate every other month – the ovaries do not coordinate alternating ovulation.

2.3.3 Luteal Phase

Regardless of whether fertilization has taken place, the corpus luteum will begin to produce progesterone, the main hormone necessary for the development of successful implantation and gestation. The corpus luteum also causes a synergistic production of estradiol, which in turn causes negative feedback on the HPO axis, decreasing both GnRH and gonadotropin excretion. If fertilization has not occurred, progesterone and estradiol levels will decline as the corpus luteum begins to involute, reaching their lowest luteal level directly prior to menstruation. The decline in progesterone causes a sloughing of endometrium, thereby signaling the beginning of menstruation and the renewal of the cycle.

2.3.4 Menstrual Cycle Effects on Sexual Function

The astute reader will notice that testosterone was not mentioned in the earlier discussion of the menstrual cycle. This is because, unlike estradiol and progesterone, testosterone levels are not dependent on cyclic hormonal variations – there is only a slight elevation in testosterone levels directly proceeding ovulation. As previously noted, the LH surge does cause an increase in gonadal testosterone production via androstenedione, and this in turn increases dopamine production in the brain. Dopamine, as will be discussed later, is one of the main excitatory neurotransmitters necessary for sexual desire. As such, an increase in dopamine often leads to an increase in sex drive. Interestingly, since the window for fertilization is very limited, this ovulatory testosterone release is more teleologic in nature as a means to continue the species and does not seem to be affected by other factors that typically regulate desire. That said, many patients admit that the only time they experience spontaneous desire is around ovulation.

Unlike testosterone, there are significant cyclic variations in both estradiol and progesterone, with the former demonstrating 200% changes in serum levels and later experiencing changes upwards of 1000% from nadirs to peaks.[17] This translates to a variety of different sexual effects, as vaginal lubrication, cervical mucus, energy levels, and even genital sensitivities are affected by these hormonal variations. Attitude to sexual activity may vary throughout the cycle as well, independent of sexual availability.[18]

Although the menstrual cycle has a significant role in sexual function, the individual hormones can affect various sexual factors regardless of cycle timing or occurrence. For example, a menopausal patient does not, by definition, have a menstrual cycle. They do, however, experience the effects of estradiol (or lack thereof) with sexual activity. As such, the individual sex hormones themselves need to be evaluated in significant detail. Understanding how these hormones interact and their effects on various receptors is paramount to practicing good sexual medicine.

2.3.5 Specific Hormones

2.3.5.1 Estradiol

Estradiol is the most potent of the estrogens, a family of steroid-based sex hormones defined by a chemical structure of 18 carbon atoms, with varying numbers of oxygen and hydrogen atoms based on the specific type. Estradiol is the estrogen responsible for the majority of the estrogenic effects in the body. The other estrogens – estrone, estriol, and estetrol – have varying degrees of bioactivity, as well as receptor binding strength. Estetrol is produced only during pregnancy, specifically by the placenta, and therefore is not considered an active estrogen outside of that specific occurrence.

In terms of sexual function, the effects of estradiol are most obvious in the female genitalia. It is estradiol that is responsible for vaginal lubrication with sexual activity, as well as the ability for the vulvovaginal tissue to expand and tolerate penetrative activity. Histologically, estradiol increases the number of superficial cells in the vulvovaginal tissue, thereby reducing tissue damage with the natural friction caused by penetrative intercourse. In menopausal patients with genitourinary syndrome of menopause, the reduction in the number of superficial cells leads to the tissue changes that accompany that condition, as well as the symptoms of painful intercourse, vaginal dryness, and atrophy of tissue. Recent research has described the effects of estradiol on the distal urethra and recommends vaginal estradiol supplementation to menopausal individuals as a means of preventing urinary tract infections.[19]

Estradiol has extragenital receptors as well, including site-specific receptors in the breast and integument, and inhibits osteoclastic activity in bone. In the brain, estradiol is produced via paracrine activity by the astrocytes and aids in creation of serotonin. It is the estradiol-serotonin relationship that is the basis of mood swings associated with low estrogen states, such as the menopausal transition as well as the later portion of the luteal phase. In addition, research into the etiology of Alzheimer's disease has found that those patients produce less estradiol, and supplementation of transdermal estradiol increased their cognitive function dramatically.[20]

BOX 2.2   ESTROGENS AND CANCER

One cannot discuss hormone therapy without discussing the correlation between estradiol and cancer. This connection is due to the Women's Health Initiative (WHI), a study of menopausal patients that began in 1991 and lasted until 2005. There are an equal number of pros and cons concerning that study, and a full review of the WHI is beyond the scope of this publication. However, it is necessary to discuss the findings of that study in terms of hormone therapy and cancer.

Prior to the WHI, hormone replacement therapy (HRT) was standard practice in the treatment of menopausal symptoms. As results (however incomplete) from that study trickled out, hormone therapy became anathema to prescribers, as the WHI demonstrated a correlation between HRT and breast cancer. Thankfully, further investigation into those results revealed inconsistencies in that data. First, the average study participant in the WHI was 63 years old, well beyond the average age of menopause. Second, the estrogen-only arm of the study demonstrated a decrease in breast cancer rates compared to placebo[21] – it was only the estrogen/progestin arm that showed a correlation between cancer and HRT. That correlation equated to an extra 8 cases of breast cancer per 100,000 menopausal women annually,[22] with a relative risk of 1.28. To put that in perspective, drinking two to four alcoholic drinks a day has a relative risk of 1.29, and daily cigarette use carries a relative risk of 1.02 to 1.32, depending on the study.[23]

Further follow-up studies have shown that transdermal estrogen replacement carries little additional risk towards developing breast cancer, and vaginally estradiol has almost no risk of breast cancer. It is postulated that the combination of the specific estrogen and progestin, as well as the extended length of time in initiating therapy from the onset of menopause, is what contributes to that slight elevation in the risk for breast cancer. Obviously, all patients who start on HRT should be counseled on risks, benefits, etc., but the public opinion that hormone therapy causes breast cancer is not as black and white as previously thought.

2.3.5.2 *Progesterone*

Much like estradiol and estrogens, progesterone is the most potent progestogen found in the human body. Progestogens are characterized by 21 carbon atoms, with varying amounts of hydrogen and oxygen atoms depending on the specific type. Progesterone, specifically, is responsible for the luteal phase of the menstrual cycle and is vitally important with the continuation of early pregnancy. In fact, prior to its "shortened" name, progesterone was known as "progestational steroid ketone," further highlighting its effects on pregnancy. This is not to say that progesterone is only necessary for reproduction, however, as it has numerous effects on sexual functioning.

Progesterone's sexual characteristics are inconsistent, and there is conflicting information regarding whether high or low levels of progesterone are better for sexual desire. One on hand, there is an increase in sex drive around ovulation – which occurs in a low-progesterone state – but conversely, many individuals experience a significant increase in desire during pregnancy, a time in which progesterone is usually at its highest. As such, there is no specific consensus on whether progesterone directly correlates with sexual desire. If it does, it is most likely due to due to its ability to increase androgen secretion through chemical conversion to 17-hydroxyprogesterone, androstenedione, and, finally, testosterone, as opposed to a direct agonistic effect on progesterone receptors.

In terms of physical manifestation, progesterone has significant effects on breast tissue in terms of lobuloalveolar and ductal development and contributes to sexual differentiation in utero.[24] There are also numerous progesterone receptors throughout the body, with significant numbers found in skin, muscle, and nervous tissue. Progesterone has a well-known protective effect on nerve tissue, and there are even some studies that have shown the benefit of progesterone supplementation in individuals who have suffered a traumatic brain injury.[25] Micronized progesterone, when taken orally, will release allopregnanolone – a metabolite with effects on allosteric modulation of the γ-aminobutyric acid type A receptor, which will produce a benzodiazepine-like effect. This explains why many individuals taking this form of progesterone at bedtime report an improvement in sleep quality.[26]

Outside of sexual medicine, the most well-known use of progesterone supplementation is in postmenopausal patients. It is well documented that those individuals on systemic estradiol therapy require progesterone to combat the proliferative effect of systemic estrogens on the endometrium. In fact, the consensus is that patients who do not have a uterus will not benefit from systemic progesterone supplementation. This idea is rife with much controversy, however, as a quick web search will demonstrate the "wonders of progesterone therapy" for all patients, regardless of the presence (or absence) of a uterus. As noted earlier, there are many progesterone receptors throughout the body, and one could argue that uterus or not, progesterone therapy may be helpful in aiding with sleep, emotional support, or other factors. The data is mixed, however, and as such, treatment should be individualized.

2.3.5.3 *Testosterone*

Testosterone is one of the main androgens, a family of cholesterol-based steroid hormones characterized by 19 carbon atoms, with varying amounts of hydrogen and oxygen atoms depending on type. Testosterone is the most common androgen in the body and is produced primarily in the gonads, with additional synthesis occurring in the adrenal glands and peripheral fat.

BOX 2.3   PROGESTINS

Synthetic progestins are often found in pharmacologic contraceptives, as well as in numerous reproductive medications to aid with regulating menstrual function. Progestins are synthetically derived from other hormones and typically have either "pro-androgenic" or "antiandrogenic" side effects, depending on their hormone of origin. Pro-androgenic progestins are more likely to cause side effects one would expect from androgens, namely acne, oily skin, and increased body/facial hair. Antiandrogenic progestins, on the other hand, are often used to treat these symptoms. Table 2.1 lists common progestins, their hormone of origin, and their androgenic properties. Of note, estranes have more androgenic effect than gonanes, and both are more androgenic than pregnanes.[27] Estranes and gonanes are the most common subgroups of progestins used in contraceptives, while pregnanes tend to be used for their endometrial effect. A notable exception to this is depo-medroxyprogesterone acetate, which is used in the injectable contraceptive Depo-Provera.

TABLE 2.1 Progestins

Pro-Androgenic	Antiandrogenic
Pregnanes – Derived from progesterone Medroxyprogesterone acetate Nomegestrol acetate	Chlormadinone acetate Cyproterone acetate Drospirenone Dienogest
Estranes – Derived from testosterone Norethindrone Norethindrone acetate Ethynodiol diacetate Norethynodrel	
Gonanes – Derived from testosterone Levonorgestrel Desogestrel Norgestimate Gestodene	

Testosterone's correlation with sexual functioning is well known.[28] In the brain, testosterone exerts dopaminergic effects, leading to both a reward-system drive to engage in sexual behavior and an excitatory effect on libido due to its connections in the mesocorticolimbic system,[29] the portion of the brain most responsible for sex drive. There is robust evidence that correlates low testosterone with low sex drive in men, but the same does not always seem to be true in female patients. In fact, high endogenous testosterone was only found to have a correlation with increased masturbation frequency in females, not in dyadic sexual activity.[30]

Outside of the sex drive, testosterone has an anabolic effect on metabolism, musculature, and bone, as well as a positive effect on mood. The later benefit is most likely due to both the earlier-mentioned dopaminergic activity and the fact that testosterone will, via aromatization, convert to estradiol, which exerts serotonergic effects on the brain. Much like any gonadal hormone, testosterone levels do decline with age, and there is a correlation between low testosterone and decreased mental acuity, especially in women.[31] As such, recent research has demonstrated possible benefits for testosterone supplementation in terms of cognition and spatial reasoning.[32]

The use of testosterone supplementation as a treatment for low libido in female patients does have some controversy. The ovaries are the main producers of testosterone, and therefore it is easy to extrapolate that decreased ovarian function would also lead to diminished testosterone levels. Whether or not this affects libido is a contested idea, especially in premenopausal patients.[33] Recently, both the Menopause Society and the International Society for the Study of Women's Sexual Health have compiled a consensus publication on the use of testosterone for the treatment of hypoactive sexual desire disorder,[34] but this publication mostly focuses on that therapy in postmenopausal patients. Is there, then, a role for testosterone supplementation in premenopausal patients? As with most topics in sexual medicine, the answer is not black and white. Local estradiol/testosterone therapy is often considered first line in treating hormonal vestibulitis,[35] and it is the author's opinion that many premenopausal patients with low serum total testosterone levels do report an improvement in symptoms such as fatigue, brain fog, and exercise intolerance, when given systemic testosterone replacement. Empiric data, as well as expert opinion, supports this practice, but the author recognizes that more formalized research on these topics should be performed before this practice would be considered standard. Regardless, supplemental testosterone does carry the risk of hyperandrogenism in the female patient regardless of menopausal status. As such, careful monitoring of testosterone therapy needs to be performed to ensure that patients do not have serum testosterone levels well beyond the upper limits of normal.

2.3.5.4 Sex Hormone–Binding Globulin

Sex hormone–binding globulin (SHBG) is a glycoprotein produced predominately in the liver. It is considered a hepatokine – a family of proteins that are secreted locally by liver cells but that have hormonal activity throughout the body. Its main function is to competitively bind to both androgens and estrogens, thereby creating a regulatory effect on those hormones by removing them from circulation. SHBG's affinity to sex hormones is as follows: DHT > testosterone > androstenediol > estradiol > estrone.[36] This means that an elevated SHBG will bind to substantially more androgens than it will estrogens, and in terms of sexual medicine, this is important for two main reasons. First, as previously stated, low androgen levels, especially testosterone, can reduce spontaneous sex drive, as well as affect sexual arousal. Second, the vestibule is rich in androgen receptors, and removing androgens from circulation may result in increased irritation, thereby leading to vestibulitis.

In the premenopausal population, the most common cause of elevated SHBG is the use of combined oral contraceptive pills containing the medication ethinylestradiol (EE). When taken orally, EE has a much greater bioavailability and is more resistant to metabolism when compared to endogenous estradiol.[37] This makes it an ideal contraceptive agent, but also makes it a relatively common culprit for androgen-related issues in premenopausal patients. There is a known polymorphism of SHBG that occurs on chromosome 17 called Rs6259 that does allow for longer circulating half-life of the protein, as well as raised serum levels.[38] This polymorphism is why some individuals will have persistently elevated SHGB even after discontinuation of EE-containing therapies. Outside of EE usage, elevated SHBG levels are often found during pregnancy, in patients with hyperthyroidism, and in women over the age of 60.[39]

Conversely, elevated androgens often occur in patients with low SHBG. This is apparent in conditions such as polycystic ovarian syndrome, hyperprolactinemia, and insulin resistance and explains why many individuals with those conditions may express phenotypic manifestations of elevated free testosterone, such as acne, hirsutism, and hair loss. Insulin resistance, in particular, seems to correlate with low SHBG and was thought historically to be due to a specific connection between the two, as both findings are often found in obese patients. Further research has determined, however, that this is most likely due to a reduction in SHBG by sugar-induced lipogenesis in the liver and not necessarily an effect of the insulin itself.[40]

Currently, there is no specific treatment for abnormal SHBG levels outside of correcting the reason for the aberration.

2.3.5.5 Prolactin

While not one of the cholesterol-based steroid sex hormones, prolactin – also known as lactotropin – can also influence sexual functioning. Prolactin is produced by the anterior pituitary in response to numerous stimuli and is mainly involved in the production of breast milk in mammals. In terms of sexual function, prolactin has an inhibitory effect on sex hormones, especially when elevated. This is especially noticeable in a patient with a prolactinoma – an often benign, prolactin-producing tumor of the pituitary – as symptoms of hypogonadism, such as amenorrhea. The exact mechanism of this suppressive effect is thought to be due to a suppressive effect on gonadotropins, although the exact mechanism is unknown. In fact, the small number of studies that have investigated this correlation noted no statistical difference in gonadotropin or even gonadal hormone levels between participants who have elevated prolactin and low sex drive – the prolactin itself remained the only significant variation.[41] Regardless, in patients presenting with low libido, a serum prolactin level is warranted as part of the initial laboratory assessment.

2.3.5.6 DHEA-S

Dehydroepiandrosterone sulfate (DHEA-S) is a conjugated androstane steroid produced solely in the zona reticularis of the adrenal cortex. Like other conjugated steroids, it is hormonally inert, as it lacks the binding ability to specific hormone receptors. It has historically been thought to hepatically convert to the prohormone DHEA, however, which does have the ability to further split into both estrogens and androgens. But there is some controversy with this theory, as a study from 2005 demonstrated that while DHEA could convert to DHEA-S, the reverse was not the same.[42]

For sexual medicine patients, serum evaluation of DHEA-S levels is not typically utilized, as the correlation between low libido and low DHEA-S is tentative at best, especially in premenopausal patients.[43,44] Some studies have demonstrated a plausible correlation between the two in postmenopausal patients,[45] but as a treatment for low sex drive, oral DHEA-S supplementation is not currently endorsed by any of the mainstream medical specialty societies. Nevertheless, it is not uncommon to see patients list DHEA-S or even straight DHEA supplements in their medication history.

2.3.5.7 Thyroid Hormones

The thyroid gland is one of the most important endocrine structures in the body. Located in the anterior neck, the thyroid regulates numerous homeostatic functions, namely metabolism, cardiovascular activity, and neurologic processes. This occurs through the following steps: thyroid-releasing hormone (TRH) is produced in the hypothalamus and causes the release of thyroid-stimulating hormone (TSH) from the anterior pituitary gland. TSH acts upon the thyroid to control the production of thyroxine (T_4). T_4 is biologically inert and only becomes active once it is converted to triiodothyronine (T_3) by removing an iodine atom. T_3 acts on receptors in target tissue and in turn regulates TSH production via a closed-feedback loop.

It has been documented that thyroid hormones affect circulating sex hormones through both specific receptors on the gonads and peripheral effects on SHBG.[46] It should be no surprise, then, that sexual dysfunction in patients with thyroid disease is very common, although often underdiagnosed.[47] For patients presenting with low drive or decreased arousal, a thorough evaluation of thyroid function is warranted, and it is imperative that the sexual medicine provider be familiar with the presentation of thyroid disease (see Tables 2.2 and 2.3).

TABLE 2.2 Hypothyroidism

Systemic Symptoms	Sexual Symptoms
Fatigue	Decreased desire
Weakness/Abnormal sensation	Decreased lubrication
Cold intolerance	Decreased genital sensation
Menstrual changes	Difficulty with orgasm
Weight gain	Decreased satisfaction
Dry skin	
Peripheral edema	
Brain fog/Decreased concentration	
Hoarseness	
Constipation	

TABLE 2.3 Hyperthyroidism

Systemic Symptoms	Sexual Symptoms
Fatigue	Decreased desire
Anxiety	Decreased lubrication
Tremor	Anorgasmia
Diarrhea	Painful intercourse
Fine hair	Decreased satisfaction
Rapid heart rate	
Weight loss	
Muscle wasting	
Exophthalmos	
Sweating	
Menstrual changes	

One must also consider the effects of thyroid antibodies on sexual function. While the data available is sparce, there is some evidence that in female patients specifically, the presence of thyroid antibodies increases the risk for sexual dysfunction.[48] The antibody to thyroid peroxidase (anti-TPO) is routinely used as a marker for Hashimoto's thyroiditis, which is the most common cause of hypothyroidism in countries with adequate iodine supplementation. To make matters more complicated, patients with Hashimoto's thyroiditis may present without typical hypothyroid features, especially in the early stages of the disease, and a routine TSH or even TSH with free T_4 may yield normal results. Anti-TPO antibodies may be elevated, however, and it is for this reason that the author recommends checking for the presence of anti-TPO antibodies, along with routine thyroid labs, in patients presenting with sexual dysfunction. Thankfully, for patients with thyroid disease–related sexual dysfunction, adequate treatment of their thyroid disorder often yields improvement in terms of sexual concerns.[49]

2.4 Conclusion

A thorough understanding of the basic endocrinologic processes that govern sexual function is imperative for the sexual medicine practitioner. As will be discussed later in this book, hormone therapy remains a staple for the treatment of multiple sexual medicine conditions, and if one does not fully comprehend the mechanisms of those treatments, it is not uncommon to have negligible results of that therapy. Furthermore, numerous medical providers tout a knowledge of "hormone replacement therapy" and often incorrectly diagnose or treat endocrinologic issues. It is not uncommon, therefore, for the sexual medicine provider to have to "clean up" after those practitioners, and as such, it is imperative to comprehend what issues those inappropriate hormone therapies may create and, more importantly, know how to address them!

2.5 Case Study

Alexis is a 25-year-old nulliparous patient who presents to the clinic complaining of low libido and painful sex. She has been sexually active for five years and admits to using condoms and combined ethinylestradiol/drospirenone oral contraceptive pills (OCPs) for contraception. She denies using any other medication, and she has a negative medical and surgical history. She states that over the past year she has noticed increasing pain with initial penetration and reports that the pain is present with any type of penetration, including inserting a tampon or undergoing a routine gynecologic exam. She states that she has also had to start using an over-the-counter (OTC) lubricant with sexual activity, as she feels that "things are super dry down there." She denies any pain with external genital stimulation and denies any abnormal discharge. Physical exam reveals an erythematous vestibule with a positive Q-Tip test. Her Skene glands are especially tender bilaterally. What is the most likely mechanism behind her pain?

  A: Early sexual activity
  B: Low testosterone from the OCP
  C: Genitourinary syndrome of menopause
  D: Reaction to lubrication

The answer is B. As stated earlier, EE causes an elevation in SHBG, thereby reducing free testosterone. As the vestibule is rich in androgen receptors, low free testosterone will often produce a hormone vestibulitis consistent with the previous findings. In addition, drospirenone is an antiandrogenic progestin, which further points towards a finding consistent with low testosterone.

Section II

Domains of Female Sexual Dysfunction

Chapter **3**

Female Sexual Desire

Function and Dysfunction

Concerns regarding sexual desire are some of the most common complaints in the sexual medicine clinic. With some studies documenting numbers as high as 48% of women with sexual dysfunction complaining of low desire,[50] it is of utmost importance to know how to diagnosis and treat this incredibly common condition. That said, patients may present reporting low desire, when in fact there are other issues at play – pain, dryness, etc. – and the desire is only a "downstream" manifestation of that primary complaint. In this chapter, the mechanism of sexual desire will be discussed in detail, building on the introduction that was provided in the previous chapter on sexual response. Variations in normal sexual desire will also be discussed, as well as concomitant pathologies that may cause low desire in those who suffer from them. Finally, individual desire disorders will be dissected, with special attention paid to key words, physical exam findings, and potential barriers to treatment. Therapies for individual disorders will be provided but will be discussed in detail in later chapters. It is also important to note that desire is an incredibly subjective thing, and one should not confuse a low number of sexual encounters or an overall low sex drive with pathology. Sexual desire disorders *only* exist in a patient who feels distressed with their sex drive.

DOI: 10.1201/9781003494522-3

3.1 Mechanisms of Sexual Desire

Sexual desire represents the drive an individual feels to engage in sexual activity, whether that be with themselves or with a partner (or partners). Colloquially, desire is synonymous with "libido," "sex drive," or even, albeit incorrectly, with "getting turned on." While the latter is more a manifestation of arousal, the former synonyms will often be used interchangeably, even in professional discourse. The term *libido* is a Latin word that means "desire" and was originally used by Freud in psychoanalytic practices. He defined libido as "energy, regarded as a quantitative magnitude . . . of those instincts which have to do with all that may be comprised under the word 'love.'" This psychic energy composed a portion of the *id*, the amalgamation of the primal driving forces of behavior. While this definition is somewhat poetic, at least in a 19th-century sense, we have since learned that libido and love are completely different entities and can occur in a fashion completely exclusionary of each other.

Psychoanalytic discussion aside, Freud was correct in that sex drive is derived from neuronal activity, namely influences of sex hormones and neurotransmitters in the nucleus accumbens (NA) of the basal forebrain. The NA and the ventral tegmental area (VTA) are active in the mesolimbic dopamine pathway, which is the portion of our brain that modulates reward. Dopamine, as hinted at in the previous chapter, is heavily influenced by testosterone, and it is from this connection that the sex drive–related propensities of androgens are derived.

In addition to neurotransmitters, sex drive is heavily influenced by the biopsychosocial triad, an idea originally postulated by Dr. George Engles in 1977.[51] In the biopsychosocial triad of desire, there is an interplay between biologic, physical factors (hormones, physiology, anatomy) as well as factors that influence the notion of desire from both an internal psychologic sense (ideas of sexuality, feelings about sexual activity) and an external environmental/social sense (relationship status, feelings about one's partner, social concepts of sexuality). If one imagines these three factors being the corners of a triangular building, it is not too hard to imagine that if one corner is removed, the building could collapse. As such, desire cannot exist without support from these ideals.

From an evolutionary standpoint, sexual desire can be equated to other "drives" necessary for the continuation of life; just as hunger propels the individual to find food, so does sexual desire make one seek sexual activity. While teleologically this makes sense, desire may also lead one to self-stimulate, especially when partnered activity cannot be found. There must therefore be another reason (or reasons) that sexual desire exists outside of pure reproduction.

As discussed in the previous chapter, numerous hormones are released during sexual activity, especially with orgasm. Two of these hormones, oxytocin and dopamine, both act on the reward center of the brain, creating an internal sense of satisfaction when released. This, in turn, reinforces the idea that sexual activity is "rewarding," thereby creating a sense of desire to engage in said activity again. Furthermore, studies have documented that oxytocin is a potent pain reliever and that the euphoric sense often achieved with orgasm may in fact provide a significant amount of pain relief.[52] This may cause individuals to desire sexual activity as a means of ameliorating discomfort.

3.2 Factors Influencing Female Sexual Desire

It goes without saying that numerous variables influence sexual desire. While an exhaustive list of such variables is out of the scope of this publication, research has demonstrated several factors that seem to be more potent in their positive effect on sex drive. Table 3.1 lists the top ten factors deemed the most efficacious in influencing desire for both dyadic and solitary sexual activity in female study participants.[53]

It is interesting to note that high levels of satisfaction in both dyadic and solitary sexual activity seem to indicate a greater likelihood of sexual desire overall. Also, while romantic love did factor into both tables, not only was it in the bottom half of factors, but it ranked higher as an influence for solitary sexual desire as opposed to partnered desire.

In contrast, the factors that contribute to lower sexual desire have not been as deeply studied, at least in terms of individual effects. While numerous

TABLE 3.1 Factors Influencing Female Sexual Desire

Factors That Influenced Dyadic Sexual Desire (Highest to Lowest)	Factors That Influenced Solitary Sexual Desire (Highest to Lowest)
Level of sexual satisfaction – participant	Masturbation in past month
Level of solitary sexual desire – participant	Desire for partnered sexual activity
Level of partner's desire towards participant	Sexual satisfaction
Level of sexual satisfaction of partner	Age
Partner's age	Relationship length
Level of partner's solitary sexual desire	Romantic love scale
Level of partner's desire in total	Infidelity online in past month
Romantic love scale – participant	College graduate
Given oral sex in the past month – participant	Masturbated in past
Level of participants desire towards solitary sexual activity	Relationship satisfaction

medical and psychologic conditions list "low sex drive" as a symptom, a definitive ranking of the causes of low desire has yet to be published. While one could theoretically apply an inverse to the factors in Table 3.1, this "negative factor" would be conjecture, not fact. Does *not* masturbating in the past month lead to lower solitary sexual desire? We cannot definitively say. This is compounded by the fact that lower desire does not necessarily represent dysfunction – an individual's degree, or lack thereof, of spontaneous desire is just that, individual. So, when does low desire become dysfunctional? In the introduction to this chapter, I stated that low desire is only a problem if it causes distress. I did not specify, however, if that distress was specifically towards dyadic or solitary sexual activity. Can one be distressed with their frequency of masturbation but content with their partnered sexual activity? Of course! It is important to keep this fact in mind as we delve into the individual desire disorders themselves, as there is not a definite delineation between the desire for partnered or solitary sexual activity. In fact, the clinician may be able to use that information to aid in the diagnosis of the disorder, as well as how to direct treatment.

Table 3.2 sets out the three female sexual desire disorders to be discussed further.

BOX 3.1   CANCER AND SEXUAL DESIRE

Generalized sexual concerns are incredibly common in women who are actively battling, or who have battled, cancer, with worldwide prevalences as high as 66%,[54] increasing to 93.5%[55] in specialized oncosexual centers. Of the four main domains of sexual dysfunction, desire disorders are overall the most frequent type of sexual concern voiced by cancer patients, with prevalences as high as 87% in individuals with breast cancer.[56] For sexual medicine providers, addressing low desire in cancer patients often involves a multidisciplinary team, as the entirety of the biopsychosocial triad is affected by the cancer diagnosis. It is not uncommon for patients to feel betrayed by their body and, in the case of breast or gynecologic cancers, feel a resentment towards their own sexual organs. Additionally, in cancers associated with human papilloma virus (HPV) infections, patients may harbor anger or frustration towards their partner, especially if they were the source of the patient's infection. Finally, the provider must remember that loss of desire may, in fact, be a symptom of another sexual concern. For instance, a patient who has undergone a mastectomy may experience low desire if they routinely orgasmed with nipple stimulation. Likewise, a patient who has undergone pelvic radiation may avoid sexual activity if they experience significant tenderness with penetration due to the radiation-induced changes to their vagina.

TABLE 3.2 Quick Reference: Female Sexual Desire Disorders

	Hypoactive Sexual Desire Disorder	Sexual Aversion Disorder	Compulsive Sexual Behavior/ Hypersexuality
Prevalence	Varies widely, increases with age	7–11%	Approximately 5% worldwide
Characteristics	Absence of spontaneous sexual thoughts or fantasies. Still able to enjoy sex. Little to no sexual initiation.	Extreme aversion to sexual contact or activity, as well as thoughts of sexual activity. Possible phobia to sexual activity.	Fixation on sexual fantasies or urges that interfere with daily life, compulsive sexual activities such as masturbation, partnered sex, or paying for sex.
Buzzwords, Key Phrases	"I would be fine never having sex again, but I still enjoy it when I have it."	"I get nauseated when I think about sex." Sex phobia. Sexual anorexia.	Loss of employment/ relationships due to sexual activity, multiple affairs.
Treatments	Psychotherapy, flibanserin, bremelanotide, Wellbutrin, stimulants, hormone therapy	Psychotherapy, CBT, desensitization, anxiolytics	Help groups, psychotherapy, SSRI, antipsychotics, mood stabilizers, naltrexone, antiandrogens
Notable Screening Exams	DSDS, FSFI, SFQ-28	FSFI	Hypersexual Behavior Inventory, multiple other surveys

3.3 Hypoactive Sexual Desire Disorder

3.3.1 Definition

Hypoactive sexual desire disorder (HSDD) is the most common sexual desire disorder.[57] It affects people of all genders and is characterized by a lack of spontaneous sexual thoughts or desires, including an absence of erotic dreams or fantasies. In relationships, individuals with HSDD may engage in sexual activity, and even enjoy it, but if asked, will often express no interest in initiating sex.

BOX 3.2

It is important to differentiate HSDD from the symptom of "low desire." A person may have a low sex drive due to illness, medication, relationship strain, or any number of potential causes and not actually have HSDD. True HSDD occurs in a biopsychosocially neutral state and will often persist if aggravating factors are removed.

3.3.2 Prevalence

Current research places the overall prevalence of HSDD in the United States anywhere between 5.4% and 13.6%, with wide variances depending on age,[58,59] As with most epidemiologic studies on sexual dysfunction, a lack of reporting by patients (or lack of diagnosis by providers) hints at a much larger prevalence than reported.

3.3.3 Etiology

The cause of HSDD is thought to be due to an inappropriate interplay between serotonin and dopamine, in what has been labeled the excitation/inhibition model.[60] In this model, dopaminergic impulses from the NA and VTA are counterbalanced by serotonin, which has an inhibitory effect on sexual desire. In a person without HSDD, these two neurotransmitters exist in harmony, with each one working appropriately to increase or decrease desire as appropriate. In the case of a patient with HSDD, however, the amount of serotonin grossly outweighs dopamine, and the end effect is a decreased level of libido. To put an analogy to this explanation, imagine that a person's sex drive is like a car. Dopamine is the accelerator pedal, and serotonin is the brake pedal. During a regular outing, the person applies the accelerator and brake when appropriate to safely drive the car. In a person with HSDD, however, the car has the parking brake on, thereby making acceleration much more difficult. This is not to say that the driver cannot overcome the parking brake and make the car move; it simply takes much more effort to do so. Likewise, one can still enjoy the ride even if the parking brake is engaged.

3.3.4 Terminology

HSDD is divided into different subtypes depending on the onset of the symptoms (lifelong vs. acquired), as well as when the distressing low desire occurs (generalized vs. situational). It is important for the clinician to establish this delineation, as correct diagnosis will allow for more targeted therapies. For instance, a patient who describes herself as someone who "always was bothered by a low drive, no matter what I was doing or who I was with" may have a different cause of their HSDD in comparison to someone who only began to have distressingly low desire after the birth of their last child.

3.3.5 Clinical Presentation

A patient with HSDD is distressed by their low sex drive. They often will include remarks in their history such as "I could never have sex again and be OK with it," or "I remember when I used to want to have sex, but something's different now." A hallmark of HSDD is that patients often still enjoy sexual activity, and many of them express frustration that their level of desire is low if they are routinely engaging in pleasurable sexual activity. Additionally, patients may not be able to recall the last time they had an erotic dream or found themselves having spontaneous sexual thoughts throughout the day.

3.3.6 Screening Tests

The Decreased Sexual Desire Screener is a five-question assessment that may be completed by either the patient or clinician that specifically aids in the diagnosis of HSDD. It may be administered prior to or during a clinical encounter and is especially helpful in delineating the specific type of HSDD present. Numerous other screening tests exist that may aid the clinician in the diagnosis of HSDD, and these will be covered in greater detail in Chapter 9.

3.3.7 Treatment

Historically, HSDD has been treated with various lifestyle modifications, as well as psychotherapy focusing on improving or ameliorating the patient's attitude towards sexual activity.[61] While this tactic for therapy remains a mainstay in terms of counseling techniques, pharmacologic therapy has also been found to be effective in treating the cause of HSDD via the previously mentioned excitation/inhibition model. Table 3.3 lists commonly prescribed medications for HSDD. Of note, two medications are specifically Food and Drug Administration (FDA) approved for the treatment of HSDD in premenopausal women: flibanserin (Addyi) and bremelanotide (Vyleesi). More in-depth discussion on those medications is available in Chapter 8.

3.4 Sexual Aversion Disorder

3.4.1 Definition

Sexual aversion disorder (SAD) manifests as a complete aversion to or avoidance of sexual contact with a partner. As with other desire disorders, this

TABLE 3.3 Treatments for Hypoactive Sexual Desire Disorder

Medication	Mechanism of Action	Dosage and Instructions	Possible Side Effects	Special Considerations
Flibanserin (Addyi)	5HT1A/5HT2A agonist/antagonist	100-g tablet qhs	Drowsiness, nausea, abdominal pain, hypotension	75% response rate in 8 weeks. If no change in symptoms after 8 weeks, D/C medication.
Bremelanotide (Vyleesi)	Melanocortin 4 receptor agonist	1.75-g pen injected SC 30 minutes prior to activity	Nausea, headache, hypertension, flushing	Effects may persist upwards of 36 hours. Prolonged usage may cause hyperpigmentation.
Bupropion (Wellbutrin)	Norepinephrine and dopamine reuptake inhibitor	Varies, at least 150 mg SR most effective	Agitation, dry mouth, anorexia	May be more effective in patients with clinical depression.
Testosterone	Binds with androgen receptors in brain, elicits dopaminergic activity	Varies	Hirsutism, acne, oily skin, virilization, elevated cholesterol, elevated hematocrit	Requires monitoring of serum testosterone levels. No current FDA-approved formulations for women in the U.S.
CNS Stimulants (Adderall, Ritalin)	Stimulates release of dopamine and norepinephrine	Varies depending on medication	Agitation, anorexia, dizziness	Habit forming, controlled substance.

aversion must also cause distress for the patient.[62] SAD is characterized by an almost phobic quality to sex, and it may be that sense of fear or anxiety that pushes the patient to be evaluated.

3.4.2 Prevalence

As with most sexual dysfunctions, the exact prevalence of SAD is difficult to determine. Various studies have placed prevalence anywhere from 7% to 11% in cis females to upwards of 17% in nonbinary individuals.[63]

3.4.3 Etiology

Unfortunately, little is truly known about the etiology of SAD. Individuals with this condition often report a history of sexual trauma – physical or emotional – or an upbringing that contained an extremely negative view of sexual contact. Additionally, the aversion to sexual activity may be due to a specific aspect of sex, such as a fear of semen, which can lead to a more generalized aversion over time.[64]

3.4.4 Terminology

SAD is characterized by either a constant, generalized aversion or one that is more situational. In patients with generalized SAD, there is not a situation or partner that changes their feelings towards sexual activity. Conversely, patients with situational SAD may have instances where the aversion is not so potent or they may be able to engage in certain activities without the same underlying degree of distress. Additionally, SAD is classified as lifelong or acquired, based on the onset of the distressing symptoms.

3.4.5 Clinical Presentation

Individuals with SAD will often present to the clinic complaining of no interest in sexual activity, either solitary or partnered, and, when asked, may divulge that they will "do almost anything" to not engage in sexual acts, including feigning falling asleep or neglecting hygiene. They may report various physical ailments when propositioned for sex, including mild symptoms such as nausea, headache, and fatigue or more severe ones such as incontinence, vomiting, or syncope. The patient with SAD may be unable to engage in nongenital sexual contact (e.g., kissing) for fear that it may lead to sexual activity or, in severe cases, may even manifest the previous symptoms when thinking about sex.

3.4.6 Screening Tests

There currently is not a specific screening test for SAD. Patients taking the Female Sexual Function Index (see Chapter 9) will routinely score low in the desire section of the test.

3.4.7 Treatments

Treatment for SAD is mainly psychologic in nature and focuses on addressing the underlying emotional issue. If the SAD is acquired or situational, couples therapy may be beneficial, as there will often be conflict in the relationship due to the condition. Anxiolytic medication has a role in helping with overt panic attacks but does not address the root cause of the disorder. There currently is not an FDA-approved medication for the treatment of SAD.

3.5 Compulsive Sexual Behavior

The author notes that compulsive sexual behavior is a controversial condition and that various resources may or may not classify it as a specific diagnosis apart from a more generalized impulse disorder. The term "sex addiction" has been applied to compulsive sexual behavior disorder, although the current Diagnostic and Statistical Manual of Mental Disorders, Fifth Edition (DSM-V) *does not list it as an addictive disorder subtype. Regardless, the author chose to include compulsive sexual behavior in the text as patients may present to the clinic complaining of symptoms colloquially associated with a "sexual addiction" or "nymphomania." In addition, it is important to not place a pathology on an individual with a high sex drive, as high sex drive by itself does not cause the degree of distress that individuals with compulsive sexual behavior report.*

3.5.1 Definition

Compulsive sexual behavior (CSB) is defined as an overwhelming preoccupation with sexual thoughts, fantasies, or behaviors that results in intrapersonal distress which cannot be voluntarily curtailed.[65] Due to the often-obsessive nature of this condition, individuals who have CSB may have significant difficulties with maintaining relationships or employment. In addition, CSB is associated with an increased likelihood of engaging in "chemsex" or paraphilias.[66]

3.5.2 Prevalence

Worldwide prevalence of CSB is estimated at approximately 5%,[67] although some studies note as many as 7% of women queried have reported distressingly high sex drives.[68] Unfortunately, due to the often troubling nature of this condition, many individuals with CSB do not seek treatment.[69] As such, the overall prevalence is most likely much higher.

3.5.3 Etiology

Currently, no specific cause of CSB has been determined. While various neurologic disorders, including traumatic brain injuries and neoplasms, have hypersexuality as a symptom, this is not the same as CSB.[70] Neuroscience and, more specifically, neuroimaging have not investigated patients with CSB with any depth, as most neuroscientific studies on sexuality come from healthy patients.

3.5.4 Terminology

CSB is divided into paraphilic and nonparaphilic subtypes. In paraphilic CBS, patients engage in compulsive sexual behavior with one of the *DSM-5*–identified paraphilias: pedophilia, exhibitionism, voyeurism, sexual sadism, sexual masochism, frotteurism, fetishism, and transvestic fetishism.[71] Nonparaphilic CSB is defined as compulsive sexual behavior that occurs outside of the realm of paraphilia, such as attending strip clubs, engaging in prostitution, or a history of repeat extramarital affairs.

3.5.5 Clinical Presentation

The key diagnostic behavior for a patient with CSB is their continued participation in sexual activities/behavior that is detrimental despite negative consequences. Similar to other impulse disorders or addiction behavior, patients with CSB may engage in sex to escape physical or emotional pain or as a means to deal with life stressors.[72] Due to the sensitive nature of this condition, individuals may not present to the clinic with CSB as their chief complaint and instead will only divulge hypersexual behavior when questioned.

Providers need to keep in mind that a clinical presentation of recurrent genital trauma or a history of multiple sexually transmitted illnesses does not equate to a diagnosis of CSB. Likewise, a sexual history with early coitarche or multiple sexual partners is not indicative of CSB. To further cloud the diagnostic process, the provider must remove any personal bias in evaluating for CSB. For example, a patient who routinely hires prostitutes on business trips may seem to exhibit behavior concerning the provider and at first glance fit criteria for CSB. If the activity does not adversely affect daily life, however, and does not cause distress, it, by definition, does not meet diagnostic standards for the condition.

3.5.6 Screening Tests

While screening tests do exist that target individuals with CSB, the majority are geared towards male patients. Additionally, due to the very sensitive and private nature of this condition, patients may not answer truthfully when screened. The Carnes Sexual Addiction Screening Test is a 25-item, self-reported screening exam that has been adjusted for both female patients and internet-based sexual activities. Additionally, the Hypersexual Behavior Inventory-19 (HBI-19) is a 19-item evaluation based off diagnostic criteria for hypersexuality as proposed in *DSM-5*.

3.5.7 Treatments

Treatment for CSB is divided into either psychotherapeutic or pharmacologic regimens. With psychotherapy, individualized counseling typically utilizes cognitive behavioral therapy techniques, identifying triggers for compulsive behaviors and reshaping the narrative around sexual activity. Alternatively, psychodynamic psychotherapy, which emphasizes addressing the core emotional dissonance causing the dysfunctional behavior, has also been shown to be effective in treating patients with CSB.[73]

While no specific FDA-approved medication for CSB exists, Table 3.4 lists the most used medications to help individuals with this condition.

It should be noted that some texts discuss the use of castration in severe cases of CSB. Obviously, this treatment is more directed at male patients, especially those with pedophilic tendencies,[74] and while inducing menopause in a patient as a means of lowering testosterone could in theory be beneficial, the risks of surgery and menopausal comorbidities outweigh the benefits in all but the most extreme cases.

3.6 Conclusion

Desire disorders are the most common type of sexual issues seen in the clinic, with HSDD alone comprising more than 10% of all types of sexual dysfunction. Despite this prevalence, desire disorders are often underreported and undertreated, as many individuals view low desire as a normal facet of aging, marriage, having children, etc. As such, it is important to tease out whether the lack of desire is problematic for the patient – low sex drive does not equal distress in most cases. In addition, one must also realize that sexual desire is incredibly dependent on environmental factors and not try and diagnosis a pathology when in fact the underlying issue is interruptions from children or uncontrollable interference. Regardless, the overall prognosis for patients with a desire disorder is a good one, as there exist many different forms of treatment for the specific condition. But, as always, a good clinician must know which treatment is correct for the patient and not prescribe problematic carte blanche therapy.

TABLE 3.4 Treatments for Compulsive Sexual Behavior

Medication Class	Specific Medications of Note	Mechanism of Action	Specific Considerations
Antidepressants	Fluoxetine described specifically, although other SSRIs are noted	Decreases urge/craving and potential preoccupation for sexual activity	Tend to be more effective in patients who have underlying depression.
Mood stabilizers	Valproic acid, lithium, carbamazepine, lamotrigine	Inhibits neuronal excitation, promotes GABAergic effects, thereby reducing craving	May be more effective in patients with bipolar disorder, not well studied in patients without bipolar disorder alone.
Antipsychotics	Benperidol	Dopamine receptor antagonist	Weak effect, may be helpful in reducing sexual thoughts.
Antiandrogens	Medroxyprogesterone acetate, cyproterone acetate	Decreases serum testosterone levels	Medroxyprogesterone 300–500 mg IM weekly; cyproterone not available in U.S.
Other	Naltrexone	Decreases euphoria/positive emotions associated with condition	Scant data, may be administered orally or intramuscularly.

3.7 Case Study

Olivette, a 30-year-old female, presents to the clinic complaining of low sex drive. She states that while she enjoys sexual activity occasionally, she honestly could "care less if I ever had it again." She states that she has been married for eight years and is in an overall "good marriage." She has two children, five and seven, and works part-time at home. Her husband is gone most of the week and is "always wanting sex when he gets home." She denies any pain with sex and can orgasm without difficulty. She currently uses condoms for contraception. She denies any medical complaints. She does not masturbate, reporting that "I find the thought of that gross – I don't want to touch myself there." She read about a medication for low sex drive on social media and would like to know if that could work for her.

What screening test would be the most beneficial to aid in the diagnosis of this patient?

A: Female Sexual Function Index (FSFI)
B: Decreased Sexual Desire Screener (DSDS)
C: Patient Health Questionnaire-9 (PHQ-9)
D: Hypersexual Behavioral Inventory-19 (HBI-19)

The answer is B. While the FSFI does look at desire, it also focuses on other aspects of sexual function, such as arousal and orgasm. The DSDS looks solely at low desire, specifically HSDD, which this patient presents with. The PHQ-9 is a basic depression screener and therefore not useful for this patient. The HBI-19 is useful for hypersexuality, not low drive.

Chapter 4

Female Sexual Arousal

Function and Dysfunction

If sexual desire is the "want" for sexual activity, sexual arousal is the "how." Current estimates place the prevalence of arousal disorders between 3.3% and 7.5% depending on age and other sexual factors,[75] but as with any sexual issue, exact statistics are hard to determine. To further complicate matters, the *Diagnostic and Statistical Manual of Mental Disorders*, Fifth Edition (*DSM-5*) combined problems with arousal and interest into one disorder, female sexual interest and arousal disorder (FSIAD), thereby making research specifically geared towards arousal more difficult to uncover. It is the author's opinion that sexual desire and sexual arousal are two separate entities and, as such, should be addressed individually. Regardless, in this chapter we will examine the mechanisms of female sexual arousal in detail, looking not only at physical causes of decreased arousal but also psychologic ones. We will discuss specific metrics for assessing arousal, although more thorough evaluations of those tests will be provided in Chapter 9. The individual sexual arousal disorders, female sexual arousal disorder and persistent genital arousal disorder/genitopelvic dysesthesia, will also be covered in detail, as will targeted therapies for both.

4.1 Mechanisms of Arousal

In its most basic form, sexual arousal is the physiologic preparation that occurs prior to sexual activity. In other words, the physical and psychological manifestations that occur in response to stimulation – be that tactile, visual, or

DOI: 10.1201/9781003494522-4

otherwise. The physiology of arousal is a mixture of autonomic and hormonal interplays, with the former being most present in the genitalia, and the latter being most evident in the circulatory system. One should keep in mind, however, that physical manifestations of arousal are not always sexual. Just as penile erections may occur spontaneously, so too can clitoral erections occur without sexual stimuli.

For physical arousal to occur, interactions involving multiple organ systems must happen almost simultaneously. For instance, to increase blood flow to the genitals, parasympathetic preganglionic innervation of the second, third, and fourth sacral nerve spaces activate paired postganglionic neurons in the genitalia, triggering vasodilation and the release of nitrous oxide in the vessels, thereby producing a tumescent state. At the same time, a release of sex hormones from the gonads, prolactin and oxytocin from the pituitary gland, and cortisol and epinephrine from the adrenal glands causes physiologic changes in multiple body systems, mimicking a sympathetic autonomic response. The result is a body that is "ready" for sexual activity, having undergone a bevy of physiologic changes in a very short time. To help simplify the physical manifestations of arousal, Table 4.1 lists

TABLE 4.1 Physical Changes with Arousal

Organ	Sexual Response	Physiologic Cause
Vulva and Vestibule	Enlargement and engorgement of labia majora and minora, clitoral erection, increased glandular secretion from Bartholin and Skene's glands	Parasympathetic innervation from sacrum triggering vasocongestion; nitrous oxide release causes vasodilation
Vagina	Lengthening, increased glandular secretion	Pelvic floor contraction, increased blood flow/ vasocongestion
Reproductive Organs	Elevation of uterus and cervix	Pelvic floor contraction
Lungs	Bronchodilation, increased respiratory rate	Release of adrenaline from adrenal glands
Cardiovascular System	Increased heart rate, increased blood pressure	Release of adrenaline from adrenal glands
Eyes	Pupillary dilation	Release of adrenaline from adrenal glands
Breasts	Engorgement, areolar enlargement	Increased blood flow, vasodilation
Skin	Flushing of skin	Cortisol production, vasodilation
Salivary Glands	Increased salivary production	Increased parasympathetic activity

specific organs and their response to erotic stimuli, as well as the physiologic cause of that response.

For the scientific evaluations of arousal, most studies on female patients have used changes in vaginal secretion – quality and quantity – as their primary endpoint metric.[76] While useful as an objective marker, some patients, especially those who have lower estrogen states, may still feel very aroused yet have diminished secretions. As such, another form of evaluation used to determine arousal is vaginal photoplethysmography (VPG, VPP), a technique in which a specialized probe uses photonic emissions to measure blood flow, thereby assessing vascular status. Although VPG is most used in the laboratory, it can be utilized in a clinical setting as well[77] and allows the clinician to evaluate for aberrant genital circulation. Newer imaging modalities such as clitoral Doppler have also allowed the sexual medicine practitioner to determine potential causes of arousal disorders,[78] but these often require specialized training for both the sonographer and interpreting physician to fully utilize.

In terms of comorbid conditions that often cause arousal dysfunction, microvascular disease (diabetes, hypertension) and neuromuscular conditions (multiple sclerosis, amyotrophic lateral sclerosis [ALS]) are the most common culprits. It should also be noted that, just like penile erectile function has recently been correlated with heart health,[79] clitoral arousal or dysfunctions can also relate to overall metabolic status.[80] As such, clinicians may also want to evaluate the patient with arousal disorders for other nonsexual conditions.

4.2 Neuropsychology of Arousal

Psychologically, arousal is an incredibly subjective term; what one may find exciting, another may find repulsive. While there have been many different models used to describe arousal – Masters and Johnson's *excitation phase*, Basson's *sexual response cycle*, and Toates's *incentive/motivation model*, to name a few – one has not been proven to be more accurate than another in truly defining what gets us "turned on." While physical signs of sexual arousal are objectively easier to measure, psychological arousal is more difficult to quantify – how do you measure emotional changes without functional magnetic resonance imaging (MRI) or other expensive technology? In addition, just as desire is affected by outside factors, so too is arousal. Pain, for instance, may cause the brain to shunt blood away from the genitalia as a means of dealing with a "threat," but can also be extremely erotic. Likewise, feelings of anxiety or shame about sexual activity can create a similar fear response in some and can conversely be arousing for others.

One must also consider the events leading up to sexual activity when evaluating a patient with arousal disorders. For many female patients, gender role expectations, perceived sexual attitudes, and levels of presexual stimuli are incredibly important for arousal to occur.[81] The idea of a "courtship" prior to sexual activity is not an uncommon need either, as many women report that intimacy, as whole, is the most important factor that leads to engaging in sexual activity.[82] As such, it behooves the clinician to inquire about the quality of the relationship, or past relationships, when patients present with arousal disorders – it is not uncommon to have a patient present with inability to become aroused only to find that their partner is gone the majority of the week or that they have not been on a date in the last year. Just as the biopsychosocial triad is paramount for issues of desire, so too is it of utmost importance for arousal.

Neuroanatomically, arousal in all forms, including sexual, is mediated by the hypothalamus. Sensory input is received and then sorted by the thalamus, which then causes a release of different neurotransmitters depending on the quality and type of the sensation. These neurotransmitters then activate the reticular activating system in the brainstem, which leads to the appropriate autonomic action and physiologic response. In sexual arousal, this system is altered by the presence of sex hormones – namely estradiol and testosterone – that also act on their respective receptors in different parts of the brain, including the amygdala (which moderates pleasure) and hippocampus (which moderates emotional processing). In addition, the interplay of dopamine and prolactin with sexual activity triggers the reward system from the nucleus accumbens, which in turn helps create the sensation of psychologic arousal and the desire to engage in sexual activity. Obviously, for patients with arousal disorders, any interruption in this system may lead to dysfunction.

Table 4.2 sets out the female sexual arousal disorders to be discussed further.

4.3 Female Sexual Arousal Disorder

4.3.1 Definition

Some controversy exists about the definition of female sexual arousal disorder (FSAD). As previously stated, FSAD was incorporated into FSIAD in the *DSM-5* despite often being considered a separate entity. Prior to the *DSM-5*, the *DSM-4* utilized the following criteria for diagnosis of FSAD:

1. Persistent or recurrent inability to attain, or to maintain until completion of the sexual activity, an adequate lubrication-swelling response of sexual excitement.
2. The disturbance causes marked distress or interpersonal difficulty.

TABLE 4.2 Quick Reference: Female Sexual Arousal Disorders

	Female Sexual Arousal Disorder	Persistent Genital Arousal Disorder/ Genitopelvic Dysesthesia
Prevalence	2.6–31.2%	1–4%
Characteristics	Objective: Decreased vaginal lubrication, decreased genital sensation, inability to maintain genital arousal during sexual activity Subjective: Decreased feeling of arousal, inability to maintain mental arousal during sexual activity	Unwanted feelings of genital arousal in nonsexual situations, may be chronic or acute, often triggered after initiation/ cessation of medication
Buzzwords, Key Phrases	"I can never have sex without extra lubrication," "I can't stay wet during sex," "I want to have sex, but my body doesn't respond"	"My genitals feel swollen a lot," "It feels like a hammer is hitting my genitals over and over," "Masturbation helps to relieve my symptoms for a little while"
Treatments	Testosterone supplementation, PDE5 inhibitors, vaginal estrogen, vaginal DHEA	Dependent on region of origin, may be multimodal
Notable Screening Exams	FSFI, SFQ-28	None

3. The sexual dysfunction is not better accounted for by another Axis I disorder (except another sexual dysfunction) and is not due exclusively to the direct physiological effects of a substance (e.g., a drug of abuse, a medication) or a general medical condition.

These criteria focused on the physical manifestations of arousal – namely vaginal lubrication and genital swelling – and did not consider genital sensation or the subjective/emotional aspect of arousal. In comparison, the *DSM-5* criteria for FSIAD requires three of the following six symptoms to be present for diagnosis:

1. Little interest in sex.
2. Few thoughts related to sex.
3. Decreased start and rejecting of sex.
4. Little pleasure during sex most of the time.
5. Decreased interest in sex even when exposed to erotic stimuli.
6. Little genital sensations during sex most of the time.

and

1. Symptoms must have lasted longer than six months.
2. Symptoms must be distressing to the patient.
3. Symptoms are not more accurately explained by a nonsexual mental health disorder, domestic abuse, medication, substance abuse, or another medical condition.

As one can see, genital changes (aside from sensitivity) are not required for the diagnosis of FSIAD, even though they were the hallmark diagnostic criteria for the *DSM-4*. This poses a problem for the clinician, as patients may report significant genital distress but do not meet the criteria for FSIAD. As such, it is the author's opinion that arousal and desire stay separate in diagnosis. Furthermore, the clinician may consider the following definition when evaluating patients for decreased sexual arousal.

BOX 4.1   FEMALE SEXUAL AROUSAL DISORDER

A condition in which there is a significant, distressing reduction in manifestations of arousal (physical and/or emotional) that has lasted longer than six months and is not better explained by a nonsexual mental health disorder, domestic abuse, medication, substance abuse, or another medical condition.

4.3.2 Prevalence

Current studies place the prevalence of this condition anywhere from roughly 2% to up 31%,[83] but some research has demonstrated results[84] much higher if vaginal lubrication (or lack thereof) is used as the defining characteristic. The author does believe that is an accurate statistic, however, as some patients with vaginal dryness are not bothered by it and therefore do not meet diagnostic criteria for the condition.

4.3.3 Etiology

The etiology of FSAD can be explained by one or more of the following occurrences:

1. Decreased hormonal status in the genitalia
2. Neurovascular changes in the genitalia
3. Neurovascular changes in the brain

As previously mentioned, hormonal deprivation in the vagina and vulva causes the tissue to withdraw and become less pliable as the ratio of parabasal cells to superficial cells grows closer to 1:1. In addition, the normally robust secretory glands in the genitalia begin to produce less transudate, and as such, vaginal dryness occurs. Likewise, vascular compromise can cause decreased secretion as blood flow to the vagina and vulva provides the main source of water to mix and form said transudate. In addition, nerve damage/underactivity in the genitalia may result in less efferent transmission of sensation, which in turn may decrease the body's natural response to tactile erotic stimuli. In the brain, injury to the hypothalamus or insula may lead to decreased sexual arousal, as the hypothalamus specifically controls the cerebral aspects of arousal.

4.3.4 Terminology

Previously, FSAD had been characterized by being genital in nature, subjective in nature, or both.[85] More recent classifications, however, have eliminated this specific terminology, as it does not fit the *DSM-V* criteria. FSAD therefore can be divided into lifelong versus acquired subtypes, as well as situational versus generalized subtypes.

4.3.5 Clinical Presentation

Patients with FSAD often present complaining of an inability to become and/or stay lubricated with sexual activity, decreased sensation with sexual activity, or, more rarely, difficulty with "feeling turned on." Patients will often still desire to engage in sexual activity and will be frustrated that "my body isn't responding like I want it to." In addition, they may report normal sensation and desire but simply be unable to appropriately lubricate without additional lubricants. Clinical examination of these patients is often inconclusive, although neurogenital testing (discussed in Chapter 8) may show decreased sensation to tactile stimulation. If possible, Doppler sonography or VPG may be useful in determining vascular status to the tissue.

4.3.6 Screening Tests

The Female Sexual Function Index (FSFI) remains the gold standard for assessing possible FSAD, specifically questions 3 to 10. The Sexual Function Questionnaire-28 (SFQ-28) is another validated, self-reported questionnaire that focuses mainly on arousal and desire.

4.3.7 Treatments (Table 4.3)

Currently, no Food and Drug Administration (FDA)–approved medications for the treatment of FSAD exist, although there are hormonal therapies approved for the treatment of vaginal dryness as a symptom. As such, off-label medication use is the standard form of treatment for patients with FSAD, and medications have been used effectively to help patients with

TABLE 4.3 Treatments for Female Sexual Arousal Disorder

Medication	Mechanism of Action	Dosage and Instructions	Possible Side Effects	Special Considerations
Vaginal Estrogen	Binds to vaginal estrogen receptors, increases number of superficial cells	Varies depending on medication	Increased discharge, localized irritation	Contraindicated with undiagnosed uterine/vaginal bleeding
Prasterone (Intrarosa)	Intracrine metabolizes DHEA into estrogens and testosterone locally	6.5-g vaginal suppository, inserted nightly before bed	Vaginal discharge, suppository is palm/coconut derived so may cause sensitivity	FDA approved for the treatment of GSM in menopausal females
Testosterone	Binds with androgen receptors in vestibule and clitoris Increases tissue growth in clitoris.	Varies, but usually topically applied to genitalia for arousal disorders	Hirsutism, acne, oily skin, virilization, elevated cholesterol, elevated hematocrit	Requires monitoring of serum testosterone levels No current FDA-approved formulations for women in US
PDE5 Inhibitors	Increased cGMP, leading to smooth muscle relaxation, specifically in vessels	Varies depending on medication Lower dose usually prescribed for female patients	Headache, nasal congestion, facial flushing, hypotension	Contraindicated with nitroglycerin-containing compounds
Bremelanotide (Vyleesi)	Melanocortin 4 receptor agonist	1.75-g pen injected SC 30 minutes prior to activity	Nausea, headache, hypertension, flushing	Effects may persist upwards of 36 hours Prolonged usage may cause hyperpigmentation.
Flibanserin (Addyi)	5HT1A/5HT2A Agonist/Antagonist	100-g tablet qhs	Drowsiness, nausea, abdominal pain, hypotension	75% response rate in 8 weeks If no change in symptoms after 8 weeks, D/C medication.
Vaginal Lubricants	Decreases friction with penetration	Available over the counter, apply prior to sexual activity	Hypersensitivity/Irritation depending on specific lubrication	Water-based lubricants may dry out faster and require multiple applications Silicone lubricants not suitable with certain devices.
Vaginal Moisturizers	Increases moisture level in vaginal tissue	Available over the counter, apply 2–3 weeks irrespective of sexual activity	Hypersensitivity/Irritation depending on specific moisturizer	Not to be used with sexual activity
Intravaginal Energy Devices	Increases blood flow, tissue collagen, and elastin	Varies depending on device, usually three or more sessions	Tissue burn, scarring, bruising, infection,	Not FDA approved, costly treatments, data is mixed on

**BOX 4.2   FEMALE AROUSAL DISORDER AND
GENITOURINARY SYNDROME OF MENOPAUSE**

Menopause, defined clinically as the absence of menstruation for 12 months or greater, is due to an overall decline in ovarian follicular activity and often manifests with a variety of physiologic changes. In terms of sexual function, the most common menopause-related change occurs in the genitalia with the development of genitourinary syndrome of menopause (GSM). GSM is characterized by vaginal dryness, painful penetration, and a decline in genital sensation, as well as frequent or recurrent urinary or vaginal infections. From a sexual medicine standpoint, GSM may be considered a type of arousal disorder, as the decline in genital hormone status leads to issues creating or maintaining genital arousal. As such, when evaluating menopause-age patients for sexual concerns, it is of utmost importance to assess for signs of hormonal deprivation in the genitalia, such as pallor, retraction, or changes in genital size. If there are questions about whether these changes are related to GSM, a Vaginal Health Index (see Appendix 4) may be performed. If GSM is diagnosed, hormone replacement, often in the form of local vaginal estrogens or Prasterone, should be considered first-line therapy. Treatment with vaginal estrogens has been shown to not only improve symptoms of genital arousal but, perhaps more importantly, to also reduce the incidence of urinary tract infections by more than 50%.[86]

decreased sexual arousal. In addition, there is some data that shows alternative therapies, such as intravaginal laser or radiofrequency energy, may promote lubrication and arousal. These treatments will be discussed in greater detail in Chapter 8.

4.4 Persistent Genital Arousal Disorder/Genitopelvic Dysesthesia

4.4.1 Definition

Persistent genital arousal disorder/genitopelvic dysesthesia (PGAD/GPD) is a condition characterized by recurring episodes of unwanted, unprovoked feelings of arousal in the genitalia. These episodes must be distressing to the patient and must also occur outside of sexual activity.

Originally described as "persistent sexual arousal syndrome (PSAS)" in 2001, the name was changed to PGAD in 2009 to eliminate any sexual connotations, with "genitopelvic dysesthesia" added to the nomenclature in 2019, as PGAD was considered more narrative in description as opposed to clinical.[87] The term restless genital syndrome has also been considered but is not currently accepted by the International Society for the Study of Women's Sexual Health (ISSWSH).

4.4.2 Prevalence

Current estimates place the prevalence of PGAD/GPD between 1% and 4% of individuals worldwide. As with other sexual medicine conditions, exact prevalence is difficult to determine due to the associated stigma. Furthermore, there is a lack of provider knowledge in terms of diagnosis, and therefore patients with PGAD/GPD may be misdiagnosed and not accounted for in the previous statistic.[88]

4.4.3 Etiology

Due to the complexity of the condition and the lack of animal models in which to study pathophysiology, the exact etiology of PGAD/GPD is unknown. It is postulated that the condition arises from a mixture of bio-psychosocial factors, often including symptoms of known medical conditions such as pudendal neuralgia or pelvic floor dysfunction. Many patients with PGAD/GPD do have catastrophization of their symptoms, and this coupled with feelings of guilt or shame seem to promote the progression of the disease.[89] There also seems to be an aberrant interpretation of afferent nerve pathways in the brain, falsely recognizing normal sensory input as noxious or distressing.

4.4.4 Terminology

According to the 2019 ISSWSH Consensus Bulletin, PGAD/GPD is broken down into five regions of origin (see Ref. 87). Those regions are:

1. Region One – End Organ
   - Clitoris
   - Vulva
   - Vestibule
   - Urethra
   - Bladder
2. Region Two – Pelvis and Perineum
   - Pelvic Floor
   - Pudendal Nerve
   - Pelvic Vasculature
3. Region Three – Sacrum, Lumbar Spine, and Cauda Equina
   - Sacrum
   - Cauda Equina
   - Lumbar Spine
4. Region Four – Spinal Cord
5. Region Five – Brain

Furthermore, PGAD/GPD is classified as continuous or intermittent depending on how often the patient experiences the symptoms, as well as lifelong or acquired based on the patient's age at onset of symptoms.

4.4.5 Clinical Presentation

Patients with PGAD/GPD may initially present with vague genital symptoms, such as recurrent pruritus, inflammation, or pain. Additionally, patients may have similar symptoms in nongenital but anatomically related areas such as the bladder, buttocks, or legs. Initially, the symptoms resolve quickly and randomly, only to return in a similar fashion. There may have been some provoking incident that starts the symptom occurrence, such as a motor vehicle accident or discontinuation of medication, but it is also common for patients to be unable to report any specific trauma or change that occurred directly prior to the onset of symptoms.

As the condition progresses, the episodes of genital dysesthesia will become more frequent and may increase in severity. This is often correlated with more psychologic distress about the symptoms, especially if the patient has sought medical care and not been properly diagnosed or treated. In addition, patients may report very aggressive descriptions of their symptoms, such as "an ice pick is being continually jabbed into my clitoris." Unfortunately, providers may attribute this extreme description as overdramatization and therefore may not take the patient's complaints seriously.

For some patients, especially if the origin of the symptom is nerve related, prolonged nerve excitation may lead to neuronal damage, and symptoms may switch from overactivity to underactivity, leading to a sensation of "deadness" or numbness in the previously sensitive area. This, in turn, may lead to further feelings of catastrophization, as patients are unable to feel any sensation in the affected tissue.

Table 4.4 lists common presenting symptoms and associated conditions for the five regions. Diagnosis and treatment algorithms for regions one to four are available online.[87]

BOX 4.4

Of special note, the diagnosis PGAD/GPD carries with it a high degree of suicidality – approaching 54% in some cases.[90] This factor is most often due to the socially isolating aspect of the condition, as well as the unrelenting nature of the disease. As such, patients who express suicidal ideations should be taken seriously and not dismissed as being "overly dramatic." As with any patient, those expressing suicidality need to be assessed for risk factors such as depression, prior suicide attempts, psychosocial stressors, or drug and alcohol misuse.

TABLE 4.4 Symptoms and Conditions Associated with PGAD/GPD Regions

	Presenting Symptoms	Associated Conditions
Region One – End Organ	Feelings of genital arousal AND one or more of the following: • Abnormal genital sensation – fullness, pruritus, pain, or burning • Painful urination • Urinary frequency • Excessive vaginal discharge • Painful intercourse • Pain with vaginal insertion	• Clitoral pathology – Keratin pearls, clitoral phimosis • Vulvar dermatoses – Lichenoid disorders, psoriasis • Vestibulitis – Hormonal or neuroproliferative • Vaginitis – Desquamative inflammatory vaginitis, chronic bacterial vaginosis • Urethral pathology – Chronic urethritis, *Ureaplasma* infection • Bladder – Painful bladder syndrome, interstitial cystitis
Region Two – Pelvis and Perineum	Feelings of genital arousal AND one or more of the following: • Pelvic pain • Pelvic floor tightness • Hip pain • Pain with defecation • Pain with sitting • Fullness in rectum • Multiple varicosities, especially on vulva, groin	• Pelvic floor dysfunction – Hypertonic pelvic floor, spastic pelvis • Pudendal neuropathy – May include one or all branches of nerve • Labral injury • Arteriovenous malformation • May-Thurner syndrome • Ehlers-Danlos syndrome/ Hypermobility • Pelvic congestion syndrome
Region Three – Sacrum, Lumbar Spine, and Cauda Equina	Feelings of genital arousal AND one or more of the following: • Abnormal sensation in genital area • Neuropathy in legs • Neurogenic bowel/bladder • Chronic low back pain • Lower extremity weakness	• Tarlov cyst • Sacral nerve root impingement • Ehlers-Danlos syndrome/ Hypermobility • Sacral trauma – Athletic injury, fall • Tethered cord syndrome • Osteoporosis
Region Four – Spinal Cord	Feelings of genital arousal AND one or more of the following: • Neurogenic bowel/bladder • Chronic low back pain • Extremity weakness or neuropathy • Balance difficulty	• Degenerative disc disease • Annular tear • Disc herniation or rupture • Osteoporosis • Previous spine surgery • Scoliosis
Region Five – Brain	Feelings of genital arousal AND one or more of the following: • Irritability • Suicidality • Tremor • Insomnia/Hypersomnia • Mood change • Mania	• Changes in medication – Specifically antidepressants, antipsychotics • Parkinson's disease • Brain tumor • Head trauma • Hyperthyroidism • Arteriovenous malformation

4.4.6 Screening Tests

Currently, there are no screening tests for PGAD/GPD specifically. That said, patients may have scores indicating distress on generalized mental health metrics, as well as screening tests for depression, anxiety, or suicidality.

4.4.7 Treatments

Treatment for PGAD/GPD is dependent on the region of origin and is often multimodal in nature. Table 4.5 lists common treatment options for the region of origin.

TABLE 4.5 Treatments for PGAD/GPD Based on Region

	Condition	Treatment
Region One – End Organ	Clitoral pathology	Removal of keratin pearls, surgical or nonsurgical release of clitoral phimosis, hormone therapy, pelvic floor therapy
	Vulvar dermatoses	Vulvar steroids, antifungal therapy, calcineurin inhibitors
	Vestibulitis	Hormone therapy, topical medication such as capsaicin, vestibulectomy
	Vaginitis	Hormone therapy, antimicrobial treatment, vaginal moisturizers, vaginal steroid medication
	Urethritis	Dietary changes, neuromodulation, antihistamines, antimicrobials
	Bladder	Dietary changes, neuromodulation, antihistamines, antimicrobials, lifestyle changes
Region Two – Pelvis and Perineum	Pelvic floor dysfunction	Pelvic floor physical therapy, chemodenervation, exercise change
	Pudendal neuralgia	Serial nerve blocks, neuromodulation, gabapentinoids, radiofrequency ablation, neurolytic surgery
	A/V malformation	Vascular stenting, embolization
	Pelvic congestion syndrome	Vascular stenting, pelvic floor physical therapy, hormonal medication

(Continued)

TABLE 4.5 *(Continued)* Treatments for PGAD/GPD Based on Region

	Condition	Treatment
Region Three – Sacrum, Lumbar Spine, and Cauda Equina	Tarlov cyst	Surgical excision, aspiration
	Disc disease	Physical therapy, pain management, TENS unit/ neuromodulation, shockwave therapy, sacral nerve stimulator
Region Four – Spinal Cord	Disc disease	Physical therapy, pain management, TENS unit/ neuromodulation, shockwave therapy, sacral nerve stimulator
Region Five – Brain	Medication-related	Change in medication dose, stop medication, consider addition of CNS sedatives
	Endocrine disorder	Appropriate medication therapy, surgical/nonsurgical management for mass effect
	A/V malformation/Neoplasm	Neurosurgical stenting, embolism, surgical resection
	Psychologic disease	Counseling, pain therapy, electroconvulsive therapy, transcranial magnet stimulation

4.5 Conclusion

While the media has done a fantastic job in normalizing arousal disorders for people with penises, the percentage of people with female arousal disorders presenting to their provider's office for specific arousal-related complaints is relatively low. This is partially due to the unfortunate, and downright dismissive, treatment of vaginal dryness as "just a factor of life." This is even more appalling when we consider that vaginal lubrication, or lack thereof, is *the* most common metric for studying female sexual arousal disorders. While there is a place for the use of lubricants in the treatment of vaginal dryness, simply suggesting that all patients who experience issues with arousal utilize exogenous lubrication as their main treatment modality is simply not correct.

As noted earlier, multiple physical and mental factors play into sexual arousal, and as such, it is important that the sexual medicine provider assess all aspects of the patient's physical and emotional state when they present with arousal issues. This holistic approach is especially necessary in patients with suspected PGAD/GPD, as they are most likely already extremely nervous and anxious discussing their symptoms with a healthcare provider. Additionally, should a patient present to their sexual medicine provider with suicidal ideation – be that from PGAD/GPD or otherwise – it is important to know what resources are available for both immediate and extended help for those patients. It may be that by asking the right questions and having an inviting, safe space, a life can be saved.

4.6 Case Study

Julia is a 56-year-old G2P2002 presents to the clinic complaining of a both-ersome feeling of fullness in her vulva. She is an avid cyclist and practices Pilates daily. She states that the sensation has been present for approximately one year and has progressed in intensity over the past month. She states that the sensation is distressing to her and is keeping her from wanting to leave the house. She also admits, in hushed tones, that it does help if she self-stimulates, but she is loath to do so. Her physical exam reveals no obvi-ous vulvar lesions, although she does admit to some hip discomfort when assuming lithotomy position. When asked, she states that she does use an over-the-counter (OTC) lubricant to help with sexual activity, as she suffers from vaginal dryness. Based on her history and exam, which of the follow-ing etiologies may be a possible cause for her complaint?

   A: Hormonal vestibulitis causing Region Three PGAD
   B: Hypertonic pelvic floor dysfunction causing Region Four PGAD
   C: Labral injury from cycling causing Region Two PGAD
   D: Female sexual arousal disorder secondary to allergy from OTC
      lubricant

The answer is C. Hormonal vestibulitis is a potential cause of Region One PGAD, not Region Three, and hypertonic pelvic floor dysfunction is a potential cause of Region Two PGAD, not Region Four. Labral injuries, often from cycling or exercise, may lead to Region Two PGAD. There is nothing in the question stem that would point towards an allergic reaction to the OTC lubricant.

Chapter 5

Sexual Pain Disorders

In 1789, Benjamin Franklin wrote, "Nothing can be said to be certain, except death and taxes."[91] The author would also like to add that pain should be considered an honorary addition to the idiom. From the burnt mouth suffered from drinking a too hot drink to the excruciating feeling of banging a knee on a table edge, pain is a fact of life. It is so common that almost 50% of all emergency room visits report pain as a chief complaint.[92] It should come as no surprise, then, that painful intercourse, otherwise known as dyspareunia, is one of the most common sexual medicine complaints. It is estimated that up to 18% of the population worldwide is affected by painful intercourse and that approximately one-fourth of women will experience painful sex during their lifetime.[93]

Traditionally, dyspareunia is classified as occurring with initial penetration, deep penetration, or both and can occur at any time during a sexual act. Patients may be very creative with their imagery regarding pain, often using descriptions such as "knife-like," "burning," "stabbing," or otherwise to describe their sensation and will often add modifiers such as locality, laterality, or radiation on their own. Nevertheless, it is of utmost importance that the sexual medicine provider be able to tease out as much information as possible about the nature of the pain, as small details that may seem unimportant to the patient may provide significant diagnostic information. In this chapter, we will evaluate the mechanisms and psychology of sexual pain, discussing not only

DOI: 10.1201/9781003494522-5

how pain happens but what it does to our brain with repetitive occurrences. We will also discuss common causes of sexual pain – vulvodynia, genito-pelvic pain and penetration disorder (GPPPD)/vaginismus, and pelvic floor dysfunction. As with female sexual arousal disorder (FSAD) and female sexual interest and arousal disorder (FSIAD), there exists some controversy over the lumping of vaginismus with GPPPD, so that will be evaluated as well. As always, specific testing for sexual pain disorders will be discussed in detail in Chapter 9.

5.1 Mechanisms of Sexual Pain

Before delving into sexual pain specifically, it behooves the provider to understand how pain is processed by the body. Throughout the body nerve endings called "nociceptors" act as sensory processing units, continually assessing the environment for three main types of distressing or "noxious" stimuli: chemical (e.g., acid, or base changes), mechanical (e.g., crushing, stretching, or cutting), or thermal (e.g., extremes of heat or cold). If the nociceptor receives information that surpasses an acceptable sensory threshold, a distress signal is sent from the nociceptor along nerve fibers to the spinal cord and then into the brain, where an appropriate response is generated. Depending on the type of stimuli, this response may take multiple forms, from withdrawing/retreating to aggressive behavior. From an evolutionary standpoint, our response to pain developed as a means of avoiding harm from potentially dangerous substances or situations. To further enforce this point, the brain can learn from previous painful experiences to modify future behavior to keep the organism "safe" by avoiding the previously painful experience. This is known as neuroplasticity and is one of the main behavioral factors that influences sexual pain (more on this in the next section).

As noted in the previous chapter on anatomy, the genital organs have a robust nerve supply, including the aforementioned nociceptors. While the body has developed multiple ways to suppress nociceptive activity during sex, it should be noted that the act of penetrative intercourse itself is a traumatic one, at least from the standpoint of the tissue. For example, with initial penetration, compression of vulvar tissue triggers mechanoreceptors in the skin which, if irritated, may transmit painful stimuli to the brain. Likewise, inadequate vaginal lubrication can lead to a burning sensation with penetration as delicate vestibular tissue is stretched and may potentially crack or fissure. Inside the vagina, deep penetration may lead to compression of tender, spasmed muscles, as in the case of pelvic floor dysfunction, or the stretching of scar tissue, reproducing the pain that is often associated with endometriosis-related dyspareunia.

Regardless, repetitive activation of the pain pathway with sexual activity will often create reflexive, protective responses, such as involuntarily shutting the legs (leg-locking) or spastic contractions of the introital pelvic floor musculature, as a means to "pull away" from pain. A similar process may occur with anticipation of pain as the body attempts to avoid the noxious stimuli. Additionally, this reaction may trigger a sympathetic autonomic response, shunting blood away from the genitalia and leading to a non-aroused state.

BOX 5.1

It is this same sympathetic response that will often trigger premature ejaculation in penises and may also contribute to the unwanted orgasm that can occur with rape or forced sexual activity.[94]

When it comes to diagnosis of sexual pain disorders, it is important to understand what parts of the genitalia are the most likely to experience discomfort. Table 5.1 lists potential causes of sexual pain depending on the location.

TABLE 5.1 Causes and Descriptors for Female Sexual Pain Disorders

Anatomic Location	Potential Cause	Descriptors, Buzzwords, Etc.
Clitoris	Clitorodynia, PGAD/GPD, pudendal neuralgia, keratin pearls	Throbbing; stabbing pain; irritation; itching
Labia	Pudendal neuralgia, PGAD/GPD, lichenoid dermatosis, vulvodynia	Itching; tearing; electricity-type pain; dull, achy pain
Vestibule	Vestibulitis, PGAD/GPD, pudendal neuralgia, pelvic floor dysfunction	Burning; stretching/tearing; knife-like; achy
Vagina – Superficial	GSM, PGAD/GPD, pelvic floor dysfunction, vaginitis	Burning; stretching; ripping; dull and achy; throbbing
Vagina – Deep	Pelvic floor dysfunction, endometriosis, adenomyosis, bowel disorders, PGAD/GPD	Achy; stabbing; knife-like; throbbing
Bladder/Urethra	Interstitial cystitis/painful bladder syndrome, pelvic floor dysfunction, UTI, PGAD/GPD	Burning with urination; frequent need to urinate; throbbing; stinging

While some patients can be very helpful in their use of descriptive adjectives, it is more common that patients will simply say "it hurts" and not elaborate too much on the type of pain unless prompted. As such, the provider should actively engage the patient in a pain narrative, eliciting answers to questions about location, provoking/relieving factors, quality of pain (stabbing, burning, etc.), radiation of pain, severity of pain (0–10 scale), and timing/occurrence of the pain. In addition, it may be helpful to ask the patient what they know about the pain process and assess how it is affecting their overall quality of life. It is all too common for a patient to present to the sexual medicine clinic with dyspareunia as their chief complaint, only to divulge after questioning that the pain is only a symptom of their true problem.

5.2 Neurobiology of Sexual Pain

While the body's innate response to physical pain is well understood, the neurobiology behind chronic pain, especially that of a sexual nature, is still being discovered. Neuroanatomically, when noxious stimuli is received from peripheral nociceptors, afferent pain signals travel to the dorsal horn of the spinal cord, up the spinothalamic tract, and terminate in the thalamus for processing (Figure 5.1).

At this point, depending on the situation in which the pain occurred, signals are then relayed to one of multiple cortical or subcortical regions,

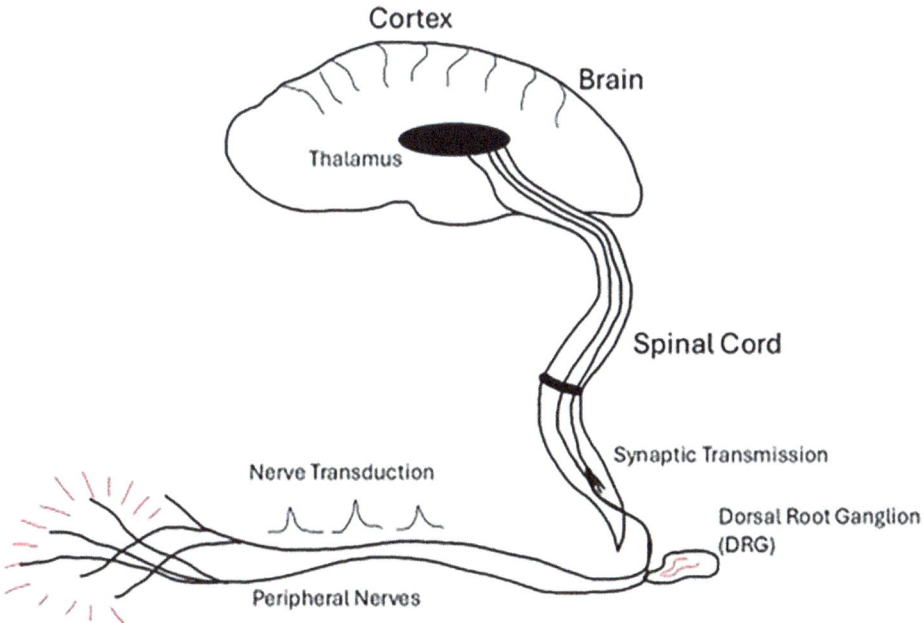

FIGURE 5.1 Pain response.

where an appropriate response to the stimulus is generated. Subjectively, our perception of pain is dependent on past experiences, context, and emotional factors and is incredibly individualized. To further complicate matters, the experience of pain is not directly tied to nociceptive activity – in other words, the sensation of pain can occur without stimuli. For example, one patient with a complex pain condition may complain of pain without obvious cause, while another may experience massive physical trauma but not outwardly appear distressed.[95]

For sexual pain specifically, the earlier process must be combined with the brain's ability to adapt to painful stimuli. This neuroplasticity has been applied to sexual pain to explain the anxiety or concern that some patients feel when sexual activity occurs, especially if there have been painful experiences in the past. Imagine an individual slamming their hand in a car door. The pain and trauma that result are not only immediate but could have lasting implications. As such, that individual will try to keep their hand safe from future smashing, perhaps by being very careful around car doors, or in an extreme case, avoiding cars altogether. The same logic applies to sexual pain – if a patient experiences pain with penetration, not only does the body physically try to escape the discomfort, but the brain creates a correlation between sex and pain. Initially, this may mean that the patient is more cautious with penetrative activity, but with repetitive exposure the patient may try to avoid sexual activity all together.

When evaluating a patient with sexual pain, it is important that the provider understand that the pain felt is not only physical but also emotional. Sexuality is a core part of the human experience, and the denial of that basic right often causes significant emotional distress.[96] While this distress may be experienced with solitary sexual activity, the addition of a partner can increase stress felt by the patient exponentially. Take, for example, the patient with dyspareunia who wants to be sexually active with a new partner. If they are hesitant to engage in penetrative activity due to concerns about pain, how will this affect their burgeoning relationship? Will their new partner be understanding, or will the partner leave them for someone else who does not have the same hesitations? While one can hope that the partner displays compassion towards the patient's condition, the unfortunate truth is that many patients feel the need to just "grin and bear it" in the face of the discomfort. This action further reinforces the association between pain and sexual activity and, if not remedied, may lead to other conditions such as vaginismus, pelvic floor dysfunction, and possible even sexual aversion. It is therefore of utmost importance that the sexual medicine provider discuss not only the physical aspects of dyspareunia with the patient but also the emotional strain that the diagnosis can bring.

Table 5.2 lists the sexual pain disorders to be discussed further.

TABLE 5.2 Quick Reference: Sexual Pain Disorders

	Vulvodynia	Vaginismus	Pelvic Floor Dysfunction
Potential Etiologies	Trauma, pudendal neuralgia, infection, dermatoses, referred pain	Trauma, social causes, anxiety, strict/religious upbringing	Trauma, childbirth, postsurgical changes, anxiety, arthralgia
Prevalence	16%	0.5–17%	10%
Characteristics	Pain localized to the external genitalia, may be generalized or provoked	Inability to tolerate penetration due to muscle spasming, may occur with nonsexual objects	Often accompanied by low back pain, urinary or fecal complaints, sensation of "bulge" in pelvis
Buzzwords, Key Phrases	Pain that worsens with sitting, "burning," or "electric" sensation along genitals	"I feel like he's hitting a brick wall," unable to tolerate tampon or speculum insertion	"I pee every time I laugh," "I can only have sex in a certain position," "My hips hurt all the time"
Treatments	Dependent on cause	Physical therapy, psychotherapy, dilator therapy, chemodenervation	Physical therapy, chemodenervation, psychotherapy, may require surgery
Notable Screening Exams	FSFI, Vulvar Pain Functional Questionnaire, vulvoscopy, Q-Tip test, vulvodoloriometry	FSFI, provocation testing	Multiple, including Pelvic Floor Distress Inventory, Pelvic Floor Impact Questionnaire

5.3 Vulvodynia

5.3.1 Definition

The word vulvodynia simply means "pain in the vulva" and is considered an umbrella term – a diagnosis that is more descriptive as opposed to specific. As such, any type of pain that occurs on the vulva may be classified as vulvodynia until a more concrete diagnosis can be made. True vulvodynia occurs in the absence of a discoverable etiology and is often very frustrating to the patient for this exact reason. According to the International Society for the Study of Vulvovaginal Disorders, vulvodynia is defined as a "chronic, vulvar pain without known etiology that lasts more than three months."[97]

5.3.2 Prevalence

An estimated 16% of women worldwide are diagnosed with vulvodynia. The condition affects women of all ages and ethnicities, with an expected lifetime prevalence of 8%. While this percentage stays constant until the age of 70, most women are diagnosed with vulvodynia between 20 and 40 years of age.[98]

5.3.3 Etiology

The exact etiology of vulvodynia is unknown, although there are multiple theories for its development. Currently, there is some debate about whether the origin of the condition is based on trauma to local tissue versus an inappropriate regional/centralized pain response. At the tissue level, trauma may lead to an appropriate nociceptive response that, with chronic occurrence or inflammation, evolves into nociceptive hyperactivity, and therefore the development of an abnormal pain response. The case of vulvodynia developing after chronic yeast infections or untreated lichen sclerosus is often given as an example of this mechanism. In addition, a deprivation in hormone levels, such as in the case of the genitourinary syndrome of menopause, or patients taking ethinylestradiol-containing oral contraceptive pills, may also lead to localized tissue irritation and the development of the nociceptive hyperactivity mentioned earlier.[99]

Conversely, patients may already exhibit inappropriate visceral/regional hypersensitivity prior to the onset of their vulvodynia diagnosis. For these individuals, alteration in the brain's pain processing ability may lead to regional hypersensitivity accompanied by other visceral reactions, such as dysuria, urinary frequency, or constipation. Furthermore, patients may ruminate on or catastrophize their condition, which further reinforces the association between vulvar sensation and pain.[100]

5.3.4 Terminology

Pain in the vulva that occurs with activity – be that sexual or otherwise – is termed "provoked vulvodynia," while pain that is present regardless is termed "generalized vulvodynia." Rarely, patients may also present with a mixed pattern. The term may be further localized into clitorodynia (for clitoral pain) and vestibulodynia (for pain in the vestibule) if the pain is isolated into one of those regions.

BOX 5.2

If an etiology for the patient's pain is found, then the diagnosis of vulvodynia changes to "vulvodynia related to/from xxx condition."

5.3.5 Clinical Presentation

The clinical presentation for patients with vulvodynia is greatly variable. Some patients may present with specific symptoms that occur at specific times, while others may only be able to provide generalized information regarding their discomfort. In addition, since vulvodynia may occur at any age, patient communication (or communication from their guardian/caregiver) regarding their specific complaints may be difficult to interpret. Regardless, pain is the basic complaint for the vulvodynia patient. Descriptors such as "burning" or "stinging" are often used if there is a neuropathic component to their pain, while the adjectives "dull" or "achy" may point towards a more vascular or musculoskeletal origin.

As expected, patients in chronic pain may also develop depression about their situation, as well as anxiety or fear regarding worsening of their pain. As such, it is important to evaluate the mental health status of patients with vulvodynia and note that patients may present with psychologic concerns as their chief complaint and, due to the sensitive/taboo nature of genital conditions, only divulge that their source of depression is vulvar pain if asked.

5.3.6 Evaluation

All patients who present with vulvar pain should undergo the Standardized Sexual Medicine Examination (SSME), preferably with vulvoscopy if available. The location and quality of the pain should be mapped, as well as notes made on whether the pain was provoked or present prior to examination. The "Q-Tip test" is a standard diagnostic test for vulvar and vestibular pain and will be covered in detail in Chapter 7. If the patient presents with symptoms concerning for infection (abnormal discharge, foul odor, pruritus, etc.), appropriate swabs should be collected and evaluated with office microscopy or by a microbiology laboratory. Hormonal testing may also be performed based off the patient's history or if the upper portion of the vestibule appears very irritated and erythematous. Should the patient complain of clitoral pain, a thorough evaluation of the clitoris should be performed, with special attention paid to the presence or absence of clitoral phimosis

---

BOX 5.3

Although seemingly inconsequential, it is the author's experience that the presence of entrapped pubic hair underneath the clitoral hood may be a cause of clitorodynia, and removal of these hairs has resulted in almost immediate reduction or resolution of pain.

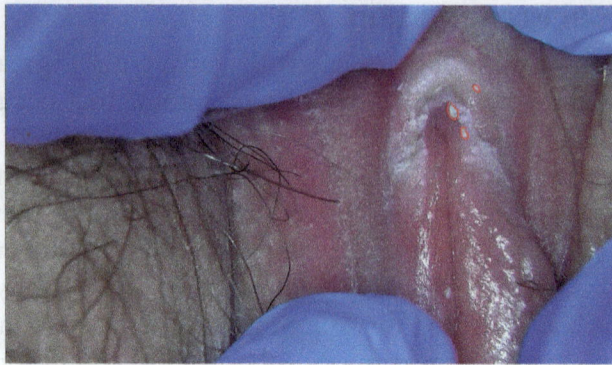

FIGURE 5.2   Keratin pearls.

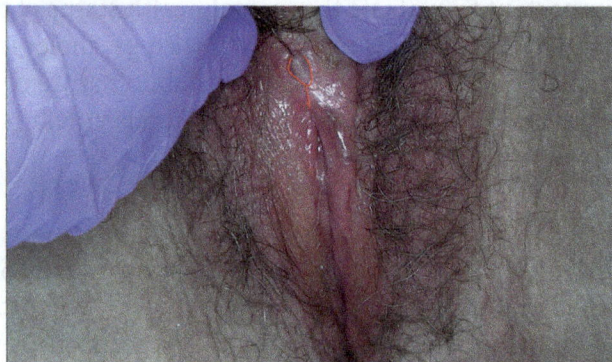

FIGURE 5.3   Clitoral adhesion.

or keratin pearls (Figures 5.2 and 5.3). Finally, vulvar skin rolling and finger percussion (Tinel's test) along the ischial spine should be performed to assess for pudendal neuritis.

A vestibular examination should be performed in a similar fashion to the vulvar exam, with special attention paid to the Skene and Bartholin glands, as well as the urethral meatus and posterior fourchette. Vulvoscopy is extremely useful in this portion of the exam, as these structures may be difficult to evaluate with the naked eye. A Q-Tip test is also recommended for this aspect of the exam.

Finally, a vaginal examination with a pediatric or small speculum should be performed and swabs taken to evaluate for the presence of infection. If necessary, 5% lidocaine cream may be applied to the vestibule to allow for reduced pain with insertion. A digital evaluation of the pelvic floor may also be performed at this time, as hypertonicity of the pelvic floor muscles may contribute to or cause the patient's pain.

5.3.7 Screening Tests

At the time of this publication, no standardized screening tests for vulvodynia have been approved by the Food and Drug Administration's Patient-Reported Outcome Guidance. That said, individual vulvar pain questionnaires are available from a variety of different sources. In addition, the Female Sexual Function Index questions 17 to 19 are geared towards dyspareunia, although not specifically towards vulvodynia.

5.3.8 Treatment

Given the multifactorial nature of vulvodynia, one specific treatment, or class of treatments, for the condition does not exist. Instead, a multimodal approach is often used to help patients manage their pain. Table 5.3 lists varying treatment modalities for patients with vulvodynia, as well as comments about specific therapies. As mentioned earlier, should an etiology for the patient's pain be discovered, treatment should be directed towards managing that condition.

TABLE 5.3 Treatments for Vulvodynia

Modality	Specific Therapies	Notes
Validation and expectation	Validation of the condition, as well as giving it a name Appropriate expectations of therapy, as well as multifaceted nature of condition Evaluation of precipitating factors for pain	The National Vulvodynia Association website has multiple resources for both patients and providers regarding vulvodynia
Lifestyle changes	Skin care: Discontinuation of irritating soaps, detergents, etc. Sexual health: Use of additional lubricants, topical numbing agents, position changes Clothing: Avoid tight, restrictive clothing Ergonomics: Cushioned seating, ice packs	Skin care: Consider daily vulvar moisturizer or barrier cream Sexual health: 2–5% Lidocaine cream to vestibule prior to sexual activity. May also use condom if male partner concerned about penile numbing
Psychotherapy	Cognitive behavior therapy Sexual counseling Couples therapy	30% reduction in symptoms in patients who undergo CBT[101]

(Continued)

TABLE 5.3 *(Continued)* Treatments for Vulvodynia

Modality	Specific Therapies	Notes
Physical therapy	Pelvic floor physical therapy Dilator therapy for desensitization Perineal massage	Be cautious when discussing Kegel exercises – for patients with tight pelvic floor, they may worsen symptoms
Pharmacologic therapy	**Antidepressants:** • SSRI/SNRI – Duloxetine, fluoxetine • Tricyclics – Amitriptyline, nortriptyline **Anticonvulsants:** • Gabapentin • Pregabalin • Lamotrigine **Hormone therapy:** • Estradiol • Estradiol/vestibular testosterone	**Antidepressants:** • Success rate for treatment in literature: 27–100%[102] • Consider side effect profile, as well as discontinuation timing **Anticonvulsants:** • 50–82% success rate[103] • Often high doses are required • Side effects may be significant at high doses **Hormone therapy:** • E2 therapy helpful in peri/postmenopausal patients, not well studied in premenopausal patients
Procedural therapy	Implantable nerve stimulators Serial local or regional nerve blocks Vestibulectomy	Vestibulectomy effective in 61–94% of cases for secondary, provoked vestibulodynia[104]

5.4 Vaginismus

5.4.1 Definition

Much like with FSIAD, controversy exists about the definition of vaginismus. In 2013, the *Diagnostic and Statistical Manual of Mental Disorders, Fifth Edition* (*DSM-5*) combined the diagnoses of dyspareunia and vaginismus into GPPPD. This decision was based on the degree of overlap between the conditions as well as similar treatment modalities. According to the *DSM-5*, to be diagnosed with GPPPD, a patient must exhibit one or more of the following criteria[105]:

1. Persistent or recurrent difficulties with vaginal penetration during intercourse
2. Marked vulvovaginal or pelvic pain during vaginal intercourse or penetration attempts
3. Marked fear or anxiety about vulvovaginal or pelvic pain in anticipation of, during, or as a result of vaginal penetration

4. Marked tensing or tightening of the pelvic floor muscles during attempted vaginal penetration

And

1. Symptoms must have lasted longer than six months
2. Symptoms must be distressing to the patient
3. Symptoms are not more accurately explained by a nonsexual mental health disorder, domestic abuse, medication, substance abuse, or another medical condition

Prior to the *DSM-5*, vaginismus was defined as a recurrent or persistent involuntary contraction of the musculature of the vagina which interfered with sexual intercourse. While this criterion does not mention fear or anxiety, it does, unlike the *DSM-5* definition, discuss the involuntary aspect of the patient's muscular contraction. In addition, the current Lamont-Pacik grading system[106] for vaginismus focuses on the patient's physical response during examination, which is objectively easier to quantify in terms of the condition's severity.

Therefore, it is the author's opinion, as well as that of other experts in the field,[107,108] that while the *DSM-5* does not list vaginismus as a specific condition, there are enough data and argument to justify its inclusion as a separate diagnosis and not simply a component of GPPPD. This is not to say that the emotional/psychologic facets of the condition that the *DSM-5* focuses on are not valid, but that they could be combined with the physical/observational findings clinicians often discover when evaluating patients.

As such, the author would like to propose providers consider this alternative definition when making the diagnosis of vaginismus:

BOX 5.4

A condition in which the muscles at the entrance of the vagina reflexively spasm in response to, or in anticipation of, pain with penetration. This spasming may be accompanied by fear or anxiety about penetration and must be distressing to the patient, last longer than six months, and not be more accurately explained by a nonsexual mental health disorder, domestic abuse, medication, substance abuse, or another medical condition.

5.4.2 Prevalence

Current research places the prevalence of vaginismus anywhere from 0.5% to 17% worldwide, with countries that identify as "more religious" or "more conservative" demonstrating higher percentages of patients with vaginismus.[109] In addition, victims of sexual or physical trauma tend have a higher risk of *developing* vaginismus.[110] While vaginismus may be diagnosed in any patient with a vagina, it is much more likely to occur in patients who have undergone puberty as opposed to prepubescent children.

5.4.3 Etiology

The exact etiology of vaginismus remains unclear, although multiple theories for its development have been suggested. As mentioned in the "Mechanism of Sexual Pain" section, pain, or the anticipation of pain, may cause the introital muscles to spasm as a means of protecting the vagina from penetration. Should continued attempts at penetration be made while the muscles are in a guarded, contracted state, neuroplastic reinforcement of penetration equating pain occurs, and vaginismus may develop. But what about individuals who have never attempted penetration? In these patients, thorough questioning will often reveal a negative emotional valence about penetration in general. They often report being told that "sex is always going to hurt," "putting something in your vagina is dirty," or some variation of these phrases. In these individuals, it may be that fear of experiencing pain or the shame or guilt associated with penetration that leads to the development of the condition.

5.4.4 Terminology

Vaginismus is classified as primary or secondary, depending on when the condition began. Patients who have always experienced a difficulty or inability to tolerate penetration are diagnosed with primary vaginismus, while those who can remember a time when penetration was not difficult or impossible are classified as having secondary vaginismus.

TABLE 5.4 Lamont-Pacik Vaginismus Grading

Grade	Clinical Findings
Lamont-Pacik Grade I	A spasm of the pelvic floor that can be relieved with reassurance, and the patient is able to relax for exam
Lamont-Pacik Grade II	A spasm of the pelvic floor that, despite reassurance, cannot be relieved, and the patient cannot relax for exam
Lamont-Pacik Grade III	Pelvic floor spasm sufficiently severe that the patient lifts her buttocks to avoid examination
Lamont-Pacik Grade IV	Pelvic floor spasm sufficiently severe the patient elevates her buttocks, retreats, and adducts her thighs (leg-lock) to avoid examination
Lamont-Pacik Grade V	Grade IV but with additional visceral response, which may include any of the following: trembling, shaking, extreme anxiety, crying, screaming, sweating, palpitations, hyperventilation, nausea, vomiting, and syncope

Additionally, vaginismus is divided into different grades of severity using the Lamont-Pacik grading[111] scale (Table 5.4).

5.4.5 Clinical Presentation

Patients with vaginismus often present complaining of an inability to tolerate vaginal penetration. Some will be able to tolerate nonsexual penetration, but the vast majority are intolerant of any type of penetrative activity, including a pelvic exam. Like all sexual concerns, patient distress is important to document, as a patient who presents with the complaints noted earlier but is not bothered by them may be the victim of coercion (which, in itself, may lead to vaginismus).

5.4.6 Evaluation

All patients presenting with vaginismus should receive the SSME as noted in Chapter 1. In addition to the SSME, the Lamont-Pacik scale may be used to further delineate the severity of vaginismus present. For some patients, provocation testing, as explained in Chapter 7, may be helpful to provoke the visible spasming of the musculature. If monitor-assisted vulvoscopy is available, it may be helpful for both the patient and/or the patient's partner to visualize the closing of the introitus to demonstrate the physical reality of the condition.

5.4.7 Screening Tests

Currently, there are no specific screening tests for vaginismus. Electromyography has been used to assess muscle tone in patients with vaginismus in the laboratory setting, but this is not the norm for clinical practice. As such, the practitioner must rely not only on patient history but also on how the patient reacts during the physical examination to accurately screen for vaginismus.

5.4.8 Treatments

Treatment for vaginismus has classically been via counseling, physical therapy, or a combination of both. The addition of vaginal trainers or dilators has also been shown to be helpful in desensitizing the introitus for penetration. In 1997 the first case report of chemodenervation with onabotulinumtoxinA (Botox) was published in The *Lancet*,[112] and since that time there has been a growing body of research demonstrating the efficacy of neuromuscular paralytic agents in the treatment of vaginismus. Currently, a multimodal approach to management seems to provide the greatest success rate in treating vaginismus, with a combination of counseling, pelvic floor physical therapy (PT), dilator work, and chemodenervation addressing all facets of the condition.[113]

5.5 Pelvic Floor Dysfunction

5.5.1 Definition

The term pelvic floor dysfunction (PFD) is a generalized clinical term that refers to disordered function of the pelvic floor muscles. Considered one of the four muscular diaphragms that exist in the human body, the pelvic floor plays an essential role in multiple tasks of daily living, such as breathing, posture, movement, defecation, and urination, not to mention sexual function and orgasm. While a complete review of the function of the pelvic floor is out of the scope of this publication, the number of patients who present to the sexual medicine clinic with symptoms related to PFD is staggering. As such, this section will focus on the sexually related aspects of PFD, namely high-tone pelvic floor musculature, and the pain-related issues that accompany that condition.

5.5.2 Prevalence

While the multifaceted nature of the condition makes it difficult to formulate an exact statistic, current estimates place the prevalence of high-tone PFD at approximately 10% worldwide.[114] As with other sexual medicine conditions, underdiagnosis of PFD is rampant, and as such the prevalence is most likely much higher.

5.5.3 Etiology

The exact etiology of PFD is not well understood and is most likely an amalgamation of various factors.[115] As such, most patients cannot recall a specific incident that precipitated their PFD. That said, risk factors for PFD are common, ranging from behavioral reasons such as inappropriate voiding techniques or stool/urine retention, to sexual trauma, to a previous history of pelvic surgery. In addition, the guarding previously mentioned in the section "Mechanisms of Sexual Pain," when occurring frequently, may lead to spasm of the pelvic floor, even at rest.

5.5.4 Terminology

From a clinical standpoint, PFD may be described based on the onset of symptoms (chronic or acute) as well as the location of the symptoms (generalized or specific). That said, most practitioners simply refer to the condition as "pelvic floor dysfunction" and do not elaborate further when discussing patient presentation. Regional language variations may include the term "high-tone pelvic floor" or "pelvic floor spasm" when describing PFD. Of note, the term "hypertonic pelvic floor" can only truly be diagnosed after observing hypertonia with electromyography (EMG).

5.5.5 Clinical Presentation

Patients with PFD may present with a variety of symptoms, including focal pelvic complaints such as pelvic pain, pressure, or stiffness, or more vague concerns such as constipation, low back pain, or urinary frequency. Depending on the location of the dysfunction, they may display an abnormal gait or posture and may show signs of discomfort when changing from seated to standing positions. When questioned about their complaints, they may describe their discomfort as "dull" or "achy" or may report a feeling of heaviness or fullness in their pelvis.

5.5.6 Evaluation

All patients being evaluated for PFD should receive the SSME as described in Chapter 1. In addition, evaluation of the pelvic floor should include the following specific testing:

- Visual inspection of the introitus for evaluation of more advanced pelvic organ prolapse. A speculum exam should also be performed to evaluate the vagina for the presence of internal organ prolapse.
- An evaluation of voluntary contraction of the pelvic floor. This may also be performed during the internal exam to assess the patient's ability to properly contract and relax the pelvic floor muscles. For patients with superficial pelvic floor spasms, it may be helpful to have them attempt to "push" against the examiner's finger to relieve discomfort with insertion.
- Individual digital palpation of the transverse perineal muscles. The examiner should pay special attention to the perineum for signs of muscular retraction/spasm.
- If posterior pelvic floor tenderness is present, digital rectal exam may be utilized to evaluate sphincter tone and posterior pelvic floor muscles, as well as to assess the coccyx, exclude rectal or anal neoplasm, and identify sources of anorectal pain, such as hemorrhoids, anal fissure, or abscess.

5.5.7 Screening Tests

Unlike the majority of sexual medicine concerns, numerous questionnaires directed at PFD exist, most of which are available for open access. As such, it behooves providers to utilize these tools to help diagnosis PFD.

5.5.8 Treatments

Treatment of PFD is often a two-fold endeavor, incorporating both relaxation therapies to relieve muscular spasm and rehabilitation exercises to

TABLE 5.5 Therapies for Pelvic Floor Dysfunction

Treatment Categories	Specific Therapies	Special Considerations
Lifestyle	Dietary changes	Avoidance of acidic foods may decrease urinary/fecal urgency associated with PFD[116]
	Counseling	Consider with long-standing history of unresponsive PFD, abuse, trauma[117]
	Weight loss	Weight loss associated with improvement in lower urinary symptoms, incontinence[118]
Medication	Muscle relaxants	Often needs multiple doses for efficacy, vaginal route more effective than oral
	Anti-inflammatory	Monitor long-term therapy GI/kidney side effects
	Hormone therapy	Helpful in patients with genitourinary syndrome of menopause
Physiotherapy	Pelvic floor PT	Considered first-line therapy for PFD Look for a certified pelvic floor physiotherapist for the best outcome
Device-Based	High-intensity focused electromagnetic therapy (HiFEM)	More data on pelvic floor strengthening and urinary incontinence treatment[119] Cost may be a barrier
	Muscle stimulator	FDA cleared for SUI, less useful for hypertonic dysfunction
Surgical	OnabotulinumtoxinA	Currently FDA approved for overactive bladder, but not pelvic floor dysfunction Research demonstrates variable success[120,121]
	Pelvic floor surgery	Limited use in high-tone dysfunction

retrain previously atrophied muscles. Table 5.5 lists common therapies for PFD, with more detail given to individual treatments in Chapter 8.

5.6 Conclusion

The evaluation and treatment of sexual pain disorders often require a collaborative approach. Referrals to physiotherapy and/or psychotherapy can be invaluable, aiding the sexual medicine provider in helping patients achieve pain-free intimacy. Additionally, it is important to understand that patients with sexual pain may feel a sense of "sexual martyrdom," disclosing that their partner's pleasure supersedes their own[122] or that "this is just how things are/should be." It is therefore of utmost importance that patients feel validated in disclosing their sexual pain and understand that pain with sex should never be the norm. Unfortunately, many patients report "medical gaslighting" when it comes to sexual pain,[123] being told by their provider to "just relax" or "drink some wine" as a means of relieving discomfort. These suggestions are almost never helpful and often worsen the patient's sense of sexual isolation. Providers should instead approach sexual pain with the same degree of thoroughness and compassion that they would if the patient were presenting with any other type of painful condition.

BOX 5.5

In certain instances, it can be very helpful to include the patient's partner in discussions and plans about the management of sexual pain. It is the author's experience that while many individuals are compassionate towards their partner's suffering, there are those who believe that sexual pain is fictitious in nature or simply a farce contrived to deprive them of sex. If possible, demonstrating that the pain felt by the patient is reproducible in the exam room with a pelvic exam may help the partner realize that the patient is, in fact, suffering.

5.7 Case Study

Christine is a 40-year-old G3P3003 who presents to the clinic complaining of worsening pelvic pain, pressure, and painful intercourse. She states that the pain is dull in quality and seems to be localized to the left side of her pelvis and vagina. She has not tried anything besides over-the-counter (OTC) medication for her pain and reports no improvement with those therapies. She is a very active individual and admits that she hurt her low back doing high-intensity exercises last year. Since that time, her pain has intensified, becoming so severe at times that she is unable to exercise due to the discomfort. When examined, she exhibits increased tone and tenderness along her left pubococcygeus and obturator internus, as well as a right and left asymmetry with voluntary contraction of the pelvic floor. A grade one cystocele is detected, but no other pelvic organ prolapse. Which of the following therapies would be the least helpful in alleviating this patient's pain?

 A: OTC lubrication during sexual activity
 B: Anterior and posterior colporrhaphy
 C: Chemodenervation of the hypertonic pelvic floor muscles with ona-botulinumtoxin A (Botox)
 D: Referral to a licensed pelvic floor physiotherapist

The answer is B. An anterior and posterior colporrhaphy is a surgery utilized to reduce pelvic organ prolapse. In patients with high-tone PFD, this procedure may worsen their symptoms. While not necessarily helpful, OTC lubricant use does not carry the same degree of risk that a surgical procedure does. Chemodenervation could be helpful in relieving the pelvic floor spasm but is not first-line therapy. Pelvic floor physiotherapy is considered first-line therapy for PFD.

Chapter **6**

Female Orgasm
Function and Dysfunction

Female orgasm has long been the subject of both scientific speculation and cultural fascination. Artistic references to orgasm have been found in multiple mediums and from multiple eras, including Ovid's *Metamorphoses*,[124] Percy Bysshe Shelley's *Fragment: Supposed to Be an Epithalamium of Francis Ravaillac and Charlotte Cordé*,[125] and Japanese *Shunga* woodblock carvings. Despite the ubiquitousness of orgasmic *Ars Erotica*, scientific research on female orgasm has lagged significantly compared to the male orgasm, with Freud reporting that female orgasm, as well as female sexuality, was a "dark continent," still waiting to be explored. Currently, this divergence in orgasmic understanding is known as the "orgasm gap" and has become a veritable hotbed of sexual medicine research. In her book, *Becoming Cliterate: Why Orgasm Equality Matters – and How to Get It*, psychologist Lauren Mintz discusses that the orgasm gap represents a type of gender discrimination resulting from "our cultural ignorance of the clitoris,"[126] as well as the fact that the female lower genital tract is often labeled colloquially as the vagina, completely disregarding the organ that most contributes to female orgasm – the clitoris. More on this later.

From a female sexual medicine standpoint, orgasmic disorders are traditionally divided into two subgroups: female orgasm disorder (FOD) and pleasure dissociative orgasmic disorder (PDOD). In addition, dysorgasmia, a condition in which patients express somatic complaints during or after orgasm, will be addressed as well. In this chapter we will discuss not only why we, as a species,

DOI: 10.1201/9781003494522-6   85 orgasm but also the physiologic and psychologic ramifications of orgasm. Since the stimulation required for an orgasm is variable, the specific statistics of "how" we orgasm will also be discussed, with special attention given towards the aforementioned orgasm gap. As always, individual disorders will be discussed in detail, as well as current diagnostic criteria and treatment options. Specific testing for orgasmic disorders will be reviewed in Chapters 7 and 9.

6.1 Orgasmic Physiology

Historically, Masters and Johnson were some of the first scientists to look at orgasm from a physiologic standpoint. In *Human Sexual Response*, they hypothesized that since arousal filled the genitals with blood and orgasm occurred after arousal, it must be the primary driving force in returning the genitals to a nonaroused state.[127] Further physiologic investigation revealed the exact mechanism for this occurrence: sympathetic innervation from the T11–L2 spinal segments leading to vasoconstriction, effectively dispersing blood from aroused/engorged tissue. In addition, this switch in autonomic control led to a reflex from the earlier-mentioned spinal cord α-motor neurons, causing involuntary muscle contractions of the pelvic floor. It is this contraction that leads to the physical sensation of orgasm, a rhythmic pelvic pulsation that often includes muscles in the pelvic floor and perianal area, as well as the movement in the uterus and cervix. Of note, a study performed in the Netherlands found that this pulsation occurred with a frequency of 8 to 13 Hz and was specific to orgasmic activity.[128] That exact frequency was unable to be reproduced when study participants attempted to fake an orgasm, demonstrating that the contractions that occur during orgasm are individualized to that specific event.

On average, a female orgasm lasts approximately 20 seconds, with additional irregular contractions occurring afterwards for varying amounts of time.[129] Directly prior to the orgasm, the lower third of the vagina contracts, while the upper two-thirds lengthens and dilates. The reason for this anatomic change is unknown, although there are myriad theories, including the idea that vaginal "clenching" will provide more stimulation to the male partner, thereby improving the likelihood that ejaculation occurs,[130] to creating a form of vaginal peristalsis, propelling semen towards the vaginal fornix.[131] The astute reader will note that these theories place female orgasm as a passive occurrence for reproduction only, effectively debasing the entire female orgasmic response and transforming the vagina into naught but a semen receptacle. With thoughts like these it is no wonder that the female orgasm remains a mystery to so many male partners!

Regardless, there is ample evidence that orgasm is a total body experience. For instance, in breast tissue, myofibroblast-related changes in the nipple-areolar complex are their greatest during orgasm, and signs of flushing and/or darkening can be detected in the skin and external genital tissue at the start of orgasm. Outside of genital changes, some individuals may exhibit involuntary vocalization during orgasm to express pleasure, while others may have uncontrolled flexion of the muscles in their extremities. In the brain, active positron emission tomography (PET) scans taken during sexual stimulation have recorded myriad changes, including a significant increase in neuron activity in multiple brain regions, such as those that affect motor function, sensory input, personality, and reward.[132]

Following orgasm, the pituitary releases large amounts of prolactin, oxytocin, and endogenous opioids, creating a sense of euphoria, as well as an overall sense of relaxation. For some individuals, the oxytocin release is strong enough to encourage partnered bonding, leading to the "postcoital cuddle." Interestingly, as testosterone is antagonistic to oxytocin, individuals with higher testosterone levels may not engage in bonding activities as often as persons with lower testosterone. This fact may be a reason for the stereotypical gender differences in postsexual activity.[133] Regardless, this postorgasmic state was coined by Masters and Johnson as the "refractory period" and historically was thought to be absent, or at least severely diminished, in women. It was believed that this difference was what allowed women to have multiple orgasms, although that research has since been questioned. In fact, a study from 2009 demonstrated that, much like their male counterpart, many female participants reported significant clitoral sensitivity following sex, as well as an associated aversion to further clitoral orgasms.[134] The fact that this study, occurring approximately 50 years later, was one of the first to refute the absence of a refractory period in women highlights the need to truly investigate differences, especially in orgasm, between the sexes.

6.2 The Orgasm Gap

From a cultural standpoint, orgasm is often considered the "goal" of sex.[135] While sexual medicine providers know this is not true, one only need look to pornography to recognize the perceived social importance of the orgasm, with more than 75% of pornographic videos showcasing ejaculation as the climax of the encounter.[136] The same cannot be said of the female orgasm, however, with the same study documenting only 18.3% of videos featuring perceived orgasmic activity from the actress(es), with the vast majority of those orgasms occurring from penis-in-vagina (PIV) activity. Does this inequity mean that we, as a society, place less importance on the female orgasm? Statistically, the answer is "yes." One only need to examine the staggering difference in the amount of research on the subject to see that the quantity of studies on female orgasm lags behind the male counterpart. Even one of the most well-known cultural references to female orgasm, the

Katz's Delicatessen scene in *When Harry Met Sally*, is based upon a man's inability to determine when a woman is faking an orgasm and not on why she needs to fake the orgasm in the first place.

In 1953 Kinsey's *Sexual Behavior in the Human Female* noted significant differences in the number of orgasms between unmarried and married American males and females. The book reported that the female subjects studied had 200 orgasms on average before marriage compared to 1500 orgasms before marriage in the male subjects. Additionally, 36% of the women queried had never had an orgasm prior to marriage, while 100% of the men studied had. Furthermore, 10% of all women studied had never had an orgasm at any point during their life.[137] This disparity was later coined the "orgasm gap" and served as a demonstration of the differences in sexual pleasure, at least related to orgasm, between heterosexual men and women in scientific literature, as well as real life. In 2022, a systemic review was published in the German periodical *Zeitschrift für Sexualforschung* evaluating all available surveys for orgasm disparities in heterosexual couples.[138] The review demonstrated that 30% to 60% of women achieved orgasm with partnered sexual activity, whereas 70% to 100% of men did, and when adjusted for contextual variables (relationship type and length, rate of sexual activity, type of sexual activity, etc.), the weighted orgasm discrepancy was approximately 30%.

So why does this orgasm gap occur? As stated in the introduction of this chapter, the orgasm gap may be due to ignorance of the clitoris. What needs to be defined in that statement, however, is which part of the clitoris is being ignored. Remember that the clitoris has both external (glans, body) and internal (crura) aspects, with the crura of the clitoris located at the entrance of the vagina. Theoretically, this could explain the thought that penetration leads to orgasm, as it is impossible to have penetrative sexual activity without some degree of clitoral stimulation. Why is it, then, that 70% of women report being able achieve orgasm from external clitoral stimulation without penetration, whereas only 18.4% can orgasm from penetration alone?[139] If the key to orgasm is penetration, as is portrayed in textbooks,[140] pornography, and even postgraduate medical training,[141] shouldn't that number be higher?

Unfortunately, it is this erroneous understanding of clitoral anatomy that has led to the view that the vagina is the main source of female sexual satisfaction. In reality, the crura, while sensitive, lack the concentrated nerve endings that are found in the external aspect of the clitoris, specifically the glans. As such, PIV sexual activity without external clitoral stimulation would be the equivalent of simply rubbing the shaft of the penis, with no attention paid to the head. While there are individuals who are able to orgasm with that type of stimulation, it is the glans that contains the highest concentration of nerves and therefore is the site most associated with orgasmic stimulation. To further reinforce this point, 92.4% of women report being able to orgasm with self-stimulation,[142] and according to a study published in 2021 that interviewed over 3000 women from across the globe about how they masturbated, 75% of the main techniques or patterns used to enhance sexual pleasure involved stimulation of the external clitoris, with the remaining 25% relying on internal clitoral stimulation via touching the entrance of the vagina.[143] It would seem, therefore, that the key to bridging the orgasm gap lies in a better understanding of both the anatomy and function of the clitoris, which makes sense, as the word clitoris is derived from the Greek word, *kleis*, meaning "key."

Table 6.1 lists the orgasmic disorders to be discussed further.

TABLE 6.1 Quick Reference: Orgasmic Disorders

	Female Orgasmic Disorder	Dysorgasmia	Pleasure Dissociative Orgasmic Disorder
Potential Etiologies	Partner factor (low foreplay, premature ejaculation, etc.), medication, hormonal deficiencies, neurovascular disorders, TBI, neoplasms	Pelvic floor dysfunction, endometriosis, PID, trauma	TBI, neoplasm, hormonal abnormalities, drug use, spinal cord injury, medication related
Prevalence	21–74%	Unknown	Unknown
Characteristics	Inability to orgasm with partnered or solo sexual activity	Somatic complaints (nausea, pain, headache) occurring during or after orgasm	Limited or lack of pleasurable sensation with orgasm. Able to feel when orgasm happens, but no enjoyment from it.
Buzzwords, Key Phrases	"I've never had an orgasm," "I can't climax"	"Having an orgasm hurts me," "I throw up after climaxing"	"I know when I've climaxed, but I don't feel anything"
Treatments	Sexual counseling, pelvic floor therapy, medication change, hormone therapy, prophylactic medications, CBD therapy	Pelvic floor physical therapy, medication, sexual counseling	Sex therapy, medication changes, pharmacologic intervention, hormonal medications, CBD
Notable Screening Exams	FSFI, Orgasm Rating Scale, (ORS) Female Orgasm Scale	FSFI, none specific to dysorgasmia	FSFI, none specific to PDOD

6.3 Female Orgasmic Disorder

6.3.1 Definition

FOD is defined as an inability, or extreme difficulty, to achieve orgasm with sexual activity. This definition is problematic, however, as the exact definition of what constitutes an orgasm is rather vague. Is an orgasm derived from clitoral stimulation the same as an orgasm that occurs with vaginal penetration? If the same patient cannot orgasm with vaginal penetration but can with clitoral stimulation, does that mean they have vaginal anorgasmia but not clitoral? To address this concern, the International Consultation on Urological Diseases created a committee to define the female orgasm, and the following classification was recommended at the 2003 International Consultation on Urological Diseases in Official Relationship with the World Health Organization in Paris[144]:

> An orgasm in the human female is a variable, transient peak sensation of intense pleasure, creating an altered state of consciousness, usually accompanied by involuntary, rhythmic contractions of the pelvic, striated circumvaginal musculature often with concomitant uterine and anal contractions and myotonia that resolves the sexually-induced vasocongestion (sometimes only partially), usually with an induction of well-being and contentment.

With that definition in mind, to be diagnosed with FOD, the *Diagnostic and Statistical Manual of Mental Disorders*, Fifth Edition (*DSM-V*) states that a patient must exhibit the following symptoms for at least six months:

1. Delayed, infrequent, or absent orgasm or markedly decreased intensity of orgasm after a normal sexual arousal phase on all or almost all occasions of sexual activity
2. Distress or interpersonal problems due to orgasmic dysfunction
3. No other disorder or substance that exclusively accounts for the orgasmic dysfunction

6.3.2 Prevalence

Statistically, the prevalence of FOD ranges anywhere from 21% to 74%, with significant variance based on geography, age, and hormone status.[145] In the United States, orgasmic dysfunction is the second most common type of sexual dysfunction, with approximately 25% of women between the ages of 18 and 59 expressing some concern with orgasm.[146] As always, the actual percentage of individuals with FOD may be higher due to a lack of appropriate screening questions by non–sexual medicine providers.

6.3.3 Etiology

Etiology for FOD is often divided into two categories: physical and psychological. As discussed previously in this chapter, aberrations in the orgasmic pathway, be that from injury, medication use, or other disease processes, may cause orgasmic dysfunction. Common culprits include neurovascular conditions such as diabetes, atherosclerosis, or stroke,[147] as well as medications that impact neurotransmitter processing, such as selective serotonin reuptake inhibitors (SSRIs) and psychotropics.[148] Pelvic floor dysfunction has been known to lead to orgasmic dysfunction, especially when dyspareunia is also present. In addition, pituitary disease is highly correlated to orgasmic dysfunction, as oxytocin plays a very important role in orgasmic function. Other abnormal hormone levels, especially low estradiol and testosterone, may also play a role in FOD, either as a cause of pain or as a cause of decreased genital sensation.[149] Psychologically, previous traumas, including rape or nonconsensual sexual activity, can affect orgasm. This is especially true if a patient were to orgasm during nonconsensual sex, as the feelings of guilt or disgust associated with that act may persist for many years.[150] Feelings of genital dissatisfaction may also play a role in FOD, and it has been hypothesized that this may be a cause for the uptick in the number of genital cosmetic surgeries over the past decade.[151]

6.3.4 Terminology

While no specific terminology for FOD exists, it may be delineated based on occurrence, with primary FOD representing patients who have never had an orgasm, and secondary FOD describing patients who have been able to orgasm in the past but now are unable to achieve climax.

6.3.5 Clinical Presentation

Patients with FOD are variable in presentation. While it is not uncommon for these patients to have other sexual comorbidities, FOD can, and does, occur on its own, especially when it is caused by medication.

6.3.6 Evaluation

As with any sexual medicine patient, a thorough evaluation of both physical and psychological factors for FOD should be performed. This includes the Standardized Sexual Medicine Examination (SSME), as well as neurogenital testing. If findings raise the suspicion that a hormonal factor may be present, serum evaluation of gonadal hormones as well as gonadotropins and prolactin may be indicated. While it is possible to evaluate serum neurotransmitter levels, this testing is often expensive and cumbersome and should only be performed in the settings of clinical research. Special attention must also be given to whether the patient's orgasmic dysfunction exists with solo stimulation, partnered stimulation, or both. If possible, concomitant evaluation with a knowledgeable therapist or sex therapist may be invaluable in aiding in diagnosis.

6.3.7 Screening Tests

As a generalized screener for orgasmic dysfunction, the Female Sexual Function Index (FSFI) does have a section devoted directly to orgasm dysfunction. In addition, the Orgasmic Rating Scale and Female Orgasm Scale are both metrics that can be used to assess patients with FOD. These metrics will be discussed in detail in Chapter 9.

6.3.8 Treatments

The mainstays of therapy for FOD are sexual counseling and directed masturbation. Sexual counseling can help address feelings of guilt or shame about orgasm and can also be helpful for treating any residual effects from previous traumas. In comparison, directed masturbation (DM) involves cognitive behavioral therapy techniques to help educate a patient about sexual anatomy, as well as feelings associated with sexual stimulation. While often thought to be more helpful in patients with primary FOD, research has also demonstrated that DM may be helpful in patients with secondary FOD, especially if the patient is uncomfortable with touching their genitalia.[152] For patients who have secondary FOD in a specific relationship, couples counseling or partner therapy can be utilized to address any underlying conflict that may be contributing to the FOD.

For patients with hormone-related FOD, especially those in menopause, hormone therapy can also be helpful in restoring genital sensitivity, as well as decreasing pain with sexual activity. Intranasal oxytocin has also demonstrated an improvement in orgasmic function for female patients.[153] Novel therapies such as platelet-rich plasma,[154] cannabinoid-based compounds,[155] or medical devices[156] show promise in treating FOD, but further research needs to be performed before these therapies become mainstay.

6.4 Dysorgasmia

6.4.1 Definition

Dysorgasmia is defined as pain that occurs during or after orgasm. While not often discussed in the literature, as the prefix "dys" means "abnormal" or "ill," the author would also like readers to consider that noxious, somatic complaints such as headache, nausea, or syncope that occur during or after orgasm should also be included in the definition of dysorgasmia.

6.4.2 Prevalence

As the vast majority of the literature on dysorgasmia focuses on male patients, the exact prevalence in the female population is unknown. In addition, some individuals who experience dysorgasmia may associate it with painful intercourse in general, further complicating the statistic.

6.4.3 Etiology

Unfortunately, due to the dearth of research on the subject, the exact etiology of dysorgasmia is unknown. When considering the physiology of orgasm, however, one may hypothesize that extremely painful pelvic floor spasms may cause pain with orgasm, as could stretching or pulling of intraabdominal adhesions, as in the case of endometriosis. Additionally, underlying infection, such as cystitis or endometritis, may also contribute to orgasmic discomfort. As for the nonpainful symptoms of dysorgasmia, autonomic variability, especially in terms of vagal-related fluctuations in blood pressure, is most likely the culprit.

6.4.4 Terminology

As with FOD, no specific terminology exists. As such, dysorgasmia may be specified based on occurrence, with primary dysorgasmia occurring in patients who always have pain or abnormal complaints with orgasm, and secondary dysorgasmia describing patients who can recall a time when they had a normal response to orgasm.

6.4.5 Clinical Presentation

Patients with dysorgasmia may present with a variety of different complaints that occur during or after orgasm. While pain is the most common of these complaints, other somatic concerns may occur as well. These concerns include but are not limited to headache, near-syncope, syncope, nausea, vomiting, or loss of bowel or bladder control. In rare instances, hyperventilation associated with orgasm may decrease seizure threshold and can induce seizure activity.[157] Rarely, a patient may present with postorgasmic "thunderclap" headaches. For these patients, consideration must be given towards the possibility of a brain aneurysm,[158] and as such, proper investigation, including but not limited to computed tomography (CT) angiography, should be performed.

6.4.6 Evaluation

Aside from the SSME, there are no specific evaluation techniques for dysorgasmia.

6.4.7 Screening Tests

Aside from the generalized orgasmic dysfunction screening in the FSFI, no screening tests/metrics for dysorgasmia exist.

6.4.8 Treatments

Treatments for dysorgasmia rely on addressing the patient's underlying complaint(s). For instance, if a patient has pelvic pain following orgasm and their exam demonstrates hypertonic pelvic floor muscles, consider referral to pelvic floor physical therapy. Occasionally, patients may require referral to cardiology, neurology, or other specialties. In this case, it is often helpful to speak directly with the provider to discuss the patient's symptoms, as information regarding dysorgasmia, especially outside of the sexual medicine world, is exceedingly rare.

6.5 Pleasure Dissociative Orgasmic Disorder

6.5.1 Definition

PDOD is a condition in which the patient is physically aware of having an orgasm but does not experience any sense of pleasure from that event. Patients with PDOD have a disconnection from the physical manifestations of orgasm and the emotional experience that accompanies it.

6.5.2 Prevalence

Current literature has not specified an exact prevalence for PDOD in female patients.

6.5.3 Etiology

PDOD is thought to occur when there is a disruption in either the release of dopamine from the nucleus accumbens or an overproduction of dopamine receptors in the brain. Remember that dopamine is the primary neurotransmitter for reward, and therefore either a decrease in production or a lack of receptor saturation may play a role in the development of the condition. As such, depression, recreational drug use – especially chronic cannabis use – low testosterone, pituitary tumors, and even age may be associated with PDOD.[159] Prescription medications that alter dopamine release, such as those used to treat Parkinson's disease, schizophrenia, or even antiemetics such as metoclopramide, may also lead to the development of PDOD. In addition, acute-onset PDOD has been associated with sensory neuropathy,[160] as well as trauma, specifically spinal cord injury.

6.5.4 Terminology

As with other orgasmic disorders, PDOD may be defined as primary or secondary, depending on the onset of the condition. In addition, the term "sexual anhedonia" has been used to describe PDOD, although PDOD is considered more specific.

6.5.5 Clinical Presentation

Patients with PDOD often present along a continuum. The subjective aspect of orgasm is individualized, and therefore patients, especially those with primary PDOD, may not report anything abnormal with their orgasm. It is not uncommon for patients with PDOD to make statements such as "I don't really understand what the big deal is with an orgasm" or "I feel something, but it's not anything like it's portrayed in the movies." For patients with secondary PDOD, the distress is much more apparent. These patients are often able to define a time when their orgasm changed – be that from trauma, medication, or otherwise.

6.5.6 Evaluation

First, the provider should seek to determine if the patient's lack of pleasure is bothersome to them. If it is, then a thorough history should be taken, with attention paid to changes in medication, cognitive function, or other feelings of depression or lack of motivation. Laboratory testing of gonadal hormones, gonadotropins, and prolactin should be performed to assess for hormonal changes. Providers should also ask about recreational drug use. Physical exam findings in patients with PDOD are often nonspecific. In addition, referral to sex therapy or to a mental health provider knowledgeable in PDOD is extremely valuable and should be performed if possible.

6.5.7 Screening Tests

Currently no specific testing for PDOD exists. Providers should consider, however, standardized depression screening, as well as screening for drug-related sexual dysfunction. As always, specific screening metrics will be described in Chapter 9.

6.5.8 Treatments

Treatment for PDOD often utilizes a multimodal approach, combining sex therapy to address psychologic and emotional factors related to the patient's condition, as well as pharmacotherapy to aid in increasing dopamine. Underlying hormonal deficiencies should be addressed as well, and hormone replacement utilized as necessary. In addition, as recreational drug use is associated with PDOD, referral to appropriate drug abuse treatment centers or providers may be helpful for certain patients.

6.6 Conclusion

The evaluation and management of orgasmic dysfunction are a vital part of sexual medicine. As the prevalence of orgasmic disorders can reach as high as 75% in some areas of the world, it is of utmost importance that the sexual medicine provider be aware of the various manifestations of orgasmic disorders and be comfortable discussing them in a nonjudgemental, approachable manner. In addition, just as patients with low desire may engage in "obligatory" intercourse to satisfy their partner, so too may patients with orgasmic dysfunction fake climaxing as a means of appeasing those they are with. To quantify this point, 59% of women admit to "faking an orgasm" at some point in their life,[161] reporting that convincing their partner that "they had done a good job" was the primary reason for the subterfuge.[162] While there is merit in positive reinforcement, faking orgasm simply to appease a partner only reinforces the notion that the patient's sexual satisfaction does not matter. Instead, if the lack of orgasm causes a problem, allowing for open lines of communication to discuss what could be different next time could be game changing. It may be that while the clitoris is the key to the female orgasm, communication is the way to bridge the orgasm gap.

BOX 6.1   NEURODIVERGENCE AND ORGASMIC DISORDERS

While not technically a medical term, neurodivergence has recently entered the medical lexicon as a way to describe a spectrum of conditions that are related to the brain's ability (or inability) to appropriately process stimuli. Examples of these conditions include autism spectrum disorder (ASD) and attention deficit hyperactivity disorder (ADHD). Individuals with neurodivergent conditions may experience abnormal sensory processing, thereby affecting their ability to achieve orgasm, or possibly finding the orgasm itself uncomfortable or even painful. Additionally, as approximately 70% of individuals with ASD have comorbid psychiatric conditions, the rate of pharmacotherapy in this population has been touted to be as high as 66%, with antidepressant and anxiolytic medications being the most common types of medication prescribed.[163] The sexual medicine provider, therefore, should be familiar with the correlations between these medications and sexual functioning. Many SSRIs have anorgasmia or blunted orgasmic sensation as a common side effect, and while changing the medication may be beneficial for the patients' sexual concerns, altering treatment regimens without first consulting the patient's psychiatric provider may be disastrous. As such, neurodivergent patients who present with sexual concerns should be approached from a multidisciplinary standpoint, with the sexual medicine provider working in tandem with the patient's regular medical team to provide the best treatment outcomes for the patient.

6.7 Case Study

Audrey is a 35-year-old patient who presents to the clinic because of a recent inability to have an orgasm. She states that she has been married for nine years and has two children via cesarean section, ages four and six. She admits to a history of endometriosis, ultimately undergoing a hysterectomy with bilateral salpingo-oophorectomy due to the severity of her disease. Because of her age, she was placed on transdermal estradiol patches, and she denies any menopausal symptoms. An SSME was performed and found to be benign aside from decreased clitoral sensitivity. Based on the patient's history, what would be an appropriate next step in the evaluation of this patient?

A: Referral to neurology
B: Transvaginal sonography
C: Referral to sex therapy
D: Serum hormone evaluations

The answer is D. Neurology referral is not indicated for this patient, as she does not have any neurologic symptoms. Transvaginal sonography would not only be invasive but also most likely not provide any pertinent information. A referral to sex therapy could be helpful in the management of her condition but does not address the physical exam findings. Due to her decrease in clitoral sensitivity, serum hormone evaluation, specifically testosterone, would be the best next step in the evaluation of this patient.

Section III

Evaluation and Management of the Female Sexual Medicine Patient

Chapter 7

Diagnostic Tests in Female Sexual Medicine

7.1 Laboratory Assessment

The history of diagnostic medicine is fascinating and worth at least a brief sojourn for all healthcare providers. Early physicians would not only use their five senses to detect changes of the lungs, heart, and menstruation but would also employ a wide range of testing techniques – some more scientifically based than others – to help aid in their diagnosis. For example, the first use of examining bodily fluids, in this case urine, for evidence of disease is attributed to the ancient Sumerians,[164] but it was Hippocrates who tied abnormal urine findings to a specific organ system, noting that since urine was the "filtrate of the four humors," that abnormalities must therefore be from the kidneys, bladder, or urethra.[165] Obviously, we have come a long way from basing disease on humoral imbalances, but much of our current understanding of pathophysiology stems from those early clinical correlations and our desire as healthcare providers to connect what we can see with what is present internally.

DOI: 10.1201/9781003494522-7

For the majority of sexual medicine patients, evaluation consists not only of a history and physical but also an assessment of possible hormonal causes for their concerns. As noted in Chapter 2, a thorough understanding of sexual endocrinology is necessary for the sexual medicine provider, and therefore it is important to familiarize oneself with standard sexual medicine laboratory studies. Additionally, some patients may present with symptoms that correlate with spinal or internal organ pathology, so it is essential that providers know what imaging modality would be the most useful for that patient. Therefore, in this chapter we will list specific laboratory and diagnostic tests and how the results of those studies may affect diagnosis. Specific testing, such as the Q-Tip test or vestibular anesthesia test, will also be addressed. Also, instead of listing every possible laboratory or imaging study, focus will be given on modalities that have high correlation to sexual medicine patients.

Finally, a note about laboratory testing in general. With menstruating patients, it is necessary to know what part of the menstrual cycle they are currently in, and while asking a patient for the date of their last menstrual period (LMP) is commonplace, it is also important to know the average length of the cycle to appropriately correlate hormonal results. For menopausal patients – especially recently menopausal ones – some hormonal variation may be present depending on the amount of peripheral hormone production sites such as the adrenal glands or fat conversion. It is also important to recognize the potential of variation between laboratory reference intervals. While it is standard practice to accept the reference interval as the 95% range of observed values in healthy patients, sample sizes to determine that value may come from as few as 20 individuals.[166] As such, it is very important for the provider to remember that, just as an abnormal result does not equal disease, so too may a normal result still be abnormal for that patient. As always, treat the patient, not the number.

BOX 7.1 STANDARD INTERVALS *VERSUS* OPTIMAL RANGE

Many practitioners feel that the standard reference intervals provided by commercial laboratories may not be the best representation of real-life patients. As such, some providers have taken to using the term "optimal" to describe a specific interval range where patients say they feel their best. The vast majority of optimal ranges are based off of clinical experience and empiric observation as opposed to specific laboratory testing, and thus optimal ranges may differ from provider to provider. The following optimal ranges are therefore based off the author's own experience, as well as the opinions of fellow sexual medicine clinicians.

Table 7.1 lists common sexual medicine–related laboratory studies. Included are standard reference intervals, as well as optimal ranges – when appropriate – for the practitioner to consider. Finally, notes about specific studies are also included.

TABLE 7.1 Laboratory Reference Studies

Study Name	Standard Reference Interval[167]	Optimal Range	Notes
Estradiol	Menstrual: 30–800 pg/mL Menopausal: less than 25 pg/mL	At least 25 for menstruating women	Goal for estradiol therapy is greater than 60 pg/mL to prevent bone loss[168]
Progesterone	Menstrual: 0.1–23.9 ng/mL Menopausal: <0.01 ng/mL	Greater than 3 ng/mL during luteal phase to detect ovulation	
Total Testosterone	Menstrual: 10–55 ng/dL Menopausal: 7–50 ng/dL	Menstrual: 25–50 ng/dL	Goal for testosterone therapy is roughly 50 ng/dL
Sex Hormone–Binding Globulin (SHBG)	Menstrual: 24.6–122.0 nmol/L Menopausal: 17.3–125.0 nmol/L	Menstrual: 50–75 nmol/L	Natural increase with age High values may correlate to OCP use Low may correlate with elevated insulin
Free Testosterone	Menstrual: 0.5–12.9 pg/mL Menopausal: 0.2–7 pg/mL	Menstrual: 2–5 pg/mL	Inversely related to SHBG Low value correlates with OCP use
Dehydroepiandrosterone-Sulfate (DHEA-S)	Menstrual: 41.2–433.2 µg/dL Menopausal: 13.9–243.7 µg/dL	Menstrual: 300–400 µg/dL	
Prolactin	Menstruating: 4.8–33.4 ng/mL Menopausal: 3.6–32.0 ng/mL		False elevation may occur if checked after breast exam
Thyroid-Stimulating Hormone (TSH)	0.45–4.5 µIU/mL	0.9–1.5 µIU/mL	
Free Thyroxine (FT$_4$)	0.82–1.77 ng/dL	At least 1 ng/dL	
Triiodothyronine (T$_3$)	71–180 ng/dL	At least 100 ng/dL	
Free Triiodothyronine (FT$_3$)	2.3–4.1 pg/mL	At least 3 pg/mL	
Thyroid Peroxidase (TPO)	0–34 IU/mL		

N.B.: For appropriate baseline evaluation, discontinue hormonal medication for at least six weeks prior to serum testing.

> **BOX 7.2 *SERUM TESTING VERSUS URINE/SALIVARY TESTING***
>
> Recent advents in commercial laboratory science have created several ways for providers to assess their patient's labs. While serum testing remains the de facto method of assessing hormones, some providers – or even patients – contract with companies to provide hormone testing through at-home urine or salivary collection. While these tests have the benefit of not requiring phlebotomy, they are not without issue. At-home urine hormone testing, for example, checks hormonal metabolites and not the specific hormone itself. Additionally, underlying kidney disease may affect filtration, and therefore can lead to inaccurate results. Conversely, salivary hormone testing, while also noninvasive, can be affected by recent oral intake, yielding similarly inaccurate findings. Obviously, it is up to the provider to determine the method in which they wish to assess for hormonal concerns.

7.2 Imaging Techniques

Historically, the science of medical imaging began in the late 19th century with the discovery of the x-ray by Wilhem Conrad Roentgen. Conventional radiography soon followed, with the 20th century seeing the advent of ultrasonography, computed tomography (CT), and magnetic resonance imaging (MRI), allowing for three-dimensional images of internal structures. Recent advances in the field have included digital technology, artificial intelligence (AI)–assisted radiologic services, nuclear imaging, and more. As the number of imaging options increases, it is important for sexual medicine providers to know which specific study to request to help facilitate their diagnosis. Discussion with a knowledgeable radiologist can be invaluable when it comes to choosing the correct type of imaging, so the author recommends discussing which specific structures need to be evaluated prior to ordering the study itself. Regardless, Table 7.2 lists common radiologic modalities used in sexual medicine, delineated by domains of sexual function. In addition, possible findings and notes about the studies themselves are also listed that may aid in diagnosis and treatment of the related dysfunction.

7.3 Specialized Tests

While the importance of a thorough history and physical cannot be understated, it is pure hubris to think that a clinician can diagnose all facets of sexual dysfunction based off those clinical activities alone. As previously discussed in this chapter, there are myriad general laboratory and imaging studies that can aid the sexual medicine provider with their differential, but, like all fields of medicine, specific tests exist to help with diagnosis. The following specialized tests have specific value in aiding the sexual medicine

TABLE 7.2 Imaging Modalities

Imaging Modality	Domain/Condition Indication	Possible Findings/Notes
X-ray		
Pelvis	• *Pain* – Vulvodynia, PFD	Most findings correlate with traumatic injury or fracture. Also consider age-related changes in menopausal sexual dysfunction. Note: For most patients, pelvic x-ray has limited use.
Ultrasound/Sonography		
Pelvic Ultrasound	• *Arousal* – FSAD, PGAD • *Pain* – PFD • *Orgasm* – Dysorgasmia	Pelvic masses (leiomyomata, tumor) can lead to pelvic pain, PFD, and even neurovascular compression if large enough. If compression is suspected, order Doppler study. Note: Transvaginal US often not tolerated in patients with vaginismus, vulvodynia, or severe PFD.
Doppler	• *Arousal* – FSAD, PGAD • *Pain* – Vulvodynia, PFD • *Orgasm* – FOD, dysorgasmia	Useful for evaluation of pelvic blood flow. Pelvic varicosities can contribute to arousal disorders, as well as pain. Decreased vascular flow associated with orgasmic dysfunction.[169] Note: Can also use on vulva or clitoris to evaluate vascular health.[170]
CT		
Abdomen/Pelvis	• *Pain* – Vulvodynia, PFD • *Orgasm* – Dysorgasmia	Possible to detect pelvic floor dysfunction due to underlying prolapse, but rarely used.[171] Most useful in evaluation for mass effect or infectious process.
Brain	• *Desire* – HSDD, SAD • *Arousal* – FSAD, PGAD • *Orgasm* – FOD	Useful for diagnosis of brain injury/CVA if acute sexual changes present. Brain neoplasm may present with sexual dysfunction as primary concern. Note: Do not use contrast if hemorrhagic CVA suspected.
CT Angiography	• *Arousal* – FSAD, PGAD • *Pain* – Vulvodynia • *Orgasm* – FOD, dysorgasmia	May be useful in diagnosis of vascular-related conditions, such as A/V malformation, in patients with sexual concerns.

(Continued)

TABLE 7.2 (Continued) Imaging Modalities

Imaging Modality	Domain/Condition Indication	Possible Findings/Notes
MRI		
Abdomen/Pelvis	• *Pain* – Vulvodynia, PFD	May be helpful in evaluation of PFD related to prolapse, as well as specific puborectalis dysfunction in specific populations.[172]
Brain	• *Desire* – HSDD, SAD • *Arousal* – FSAD, PGAD • *Orgasm* – FOD, PDOD	Functional brain MRI has significant potential to aid in diagnosis of sexual dysfunction, but still in infancy.[173] Able to assess for brain neoplasm, especially pituitary, if hormonal cause likely. Consider brain imaging if sexual dysfunction in addition to new-onset headache, visual changes. Note: Request specific pituitary imaging study for pituitary lesion.
Spine	• *Arousal* – FSAD, PGAD • *Pain* – Vulvodynia, PFD • *Orgasm* – FOD, dysorgasmia	Able to evaluate for disc- and cord-related changes, such as annular tear, nerve impingement, or tethered cord syndrome. Sacral Tarlov cysts specifically correlate to PGAD symptoms. Demyelination of spinal cord correlated to sexual dysfunction.[174] Note: May need to have radiologist specially report Tarlov cyst, as often considered incidental, nonpathologic finding.
MRA		
	• *Arousal* – FSAD, PGAD • *Pain* – Vulvodynia • *Orgasm* – FOD, dysorgasmia	Mostly performed in research setting.[175] Similar findings to CTA, but noninvasive.

provider narrow down their list of possible etiologies. Of note, not all clinics are equipped to perform these tests, so if other, nonspecialized evaluations are inconclusive, it is advised to refer the patient to a specific sexual medicine center (see Appendix 1).

7.3.1 Neurogenital Testing

Neurogenital testing[176] encompasses not only the evaluation of possible nerve-related compromise in the genitalia but is also used to determine the presence of possible spinal cord/brain involvement. It is of particular use in the evaluation of persistent genital arousal disorder (PGAD), but also has some application for patients with symptoms suspicious for pudendal neuralgia. Neurogenital testing is divided into the three categories noted next.

7.3.1.1 Qualitative Sensory Nerve Testing

Qualitative sensory nerve testing (QST) involves testing both myelinate Aβ fibers in the external genitalia and perianal region using vibration, as well as smaller Aδ fibers (hot sensation) and unmyelinated c fibers (cold sensation) using temperature change. While large sexual medicine centers may have dedicated biothesiometry devices, a small, vibrating massager can be used to evaluate the Aβ fibers, and an obstetric swab stick placed in alternating warm and cold water can be used to evaluate temperature detection. An inappropriate response – such as inability to distinguish between hot and cold – denotes possible derangement of the S2–S4 nerve space or the possible presence of demyelinating disorders such as multiple sclerosis.

7.3.1.2 Sacral Dermatome Testing

Sacral dermatome testing is performed with the patient in prone position, using either a biothesiometer or a vibrational device to map out the specific sacral dermatomes. Vibration detection is then compared between sides. Significant variation in detection from one side compared to the other correlates with possible laterality to a spinal or neurologic lesion.

7.3.1.3 Bulbocavernosus Reflex Latency

Bulbocavernosus (BC) reflex latency testing requires electromyography (EMG) and is used to assess for contraction of the BC reflex when vibratory stimulation is applied to the right and left sides of the glans clitoris. Absence of contraction denotes an interruption in the reflex arc of the BC and may represent demyelination or nerve trauma. In some patients, visual inspection of the vestibule or the external anal sphincter without EMG may demonstrate an involuntary contraction with stimulation of the clitoris, but the lack of an obvious contraction does not necessarily mean that a neurologic defect is present.

Table 7.3 lists possible outcomes for neurogenital testing by region and modality.

7.3.2 Photoplethysmography

The science of photoplethysmography utilizes light to detect vascular changes in a tissue bed. Most practitioners are familiar with photoplethysmography via the common digital pulse oximeter, a device frequently used

TABLE 7.3 Neurogenital Testing

Anatomic Location	Qualitative Sensory Nerve Test	Sacral Dermatome Testing	Bulbocavernosus Reflex Latency
External Genitalia	Abnormal	Normal	Abnormal
Internal Pelvis	Abnormal	Normal	Abnormal
Sacrum/Cauda Equina	Abnormal	Abnormal	Abnormal
Spine	Abnormal	Abnormal	Normal
Brain	Abnormal	Abnormal	Normal

to gather pulse rate as well as oxygenation. For sexual medicine purposes, variations of this technology exist in the form of both clitoral and vaginal photoplethysmographs. These devices are used to detect changes in blood flow associated with arousal and can also be helpful in determining changes in pulse amplitude due to sexual inhibition.[177] Vaginal photoplethysmography, specifically, can also differentiate between an increase in blood flow due to anxiety versus an increase due to sexual stimulation.[178] This may be helpful in evaluating patients who present stating that they can feel aroused emotionally but are unable to become aroused physically.

7.3.3 Pudendal Nerve Block

The pudendal nerve block[179] is an anesthetic technique in which a local anesthetic agent – usually lidocaine or bupivacaine – is injected into or around the pudendal nerve sheath. While the procedure has a rich history in the realm of obstetrics, sexual medicine providers may utilize this block to help aid in the diagnosis of specific causes of vulvodynia, PGAD, or dyspareunia in general. The pudendal nerve may be accessed a variety of different ways, utilizing transvaginal, perineal, or perirectal approaches. Regardless of which approach is used, the goal of the procedure is to inject anesthetic agent(s) and/or steroids into the lesser sciatic foramen, which is located 1 cm inferomedial to the attachment of the sacrospinous ligament to the ischial spine. This allows for the medication to bathe the nerve and produce the desired anesthetic effect. For most female patients, a transvaginal pudendal nerve block is preferred and is discussed in detail in Chapter 8.

7.3.4 Vaginal Valium Trial

Diazepam (Valium) is a member of the benzodiazepine family and has been used for a variety of different indications, including anxiety, alcohol withdrawal syndrome, restless leg syndrome, and muscle relaxation. It can be administered orally, vaginally, rectally, intravenously, or intramuscularly and has a variable onset of action depending on the route of administration.

For the sexual medicine provider, its use as a muscle relaxant is well documented,[180] with a variety of practitioners prescribing vaginal tablets or suppositories for on-demand treatment for pelvic floor dysfunction and dyspareunia. Its pharmacokinetics, however, demonstrate a low peak serum concentration of 31 ng/mL occurring 3.1 hours after insertion, with a lengthy half-life of 82 hours.[181] As such, patients may not see much benefit with an as-needed use of the medication but will instead demonstrate improvement in symptoms if scheduled insertion occurs.

Due to the possibility of side effects, however, as well as the addictive potential of benzodiazepines, it is the belief of the author that vaginal Valium should be used as a diagnostic test and not as a treatment. The vaginal Valium trial (VVT), therefore, is a diagnostic modality that involves prescribing nine 10 mg Valium tablets and having the patient insert one tablet vaginally or rectally every eight hours for three days. Due to the half-life of the medication, the cumulative therapeutic effect of the trial is most noticed after the third day of the series, with a positive VVT being reported as a roughly 20% to 30% reduction in pain or spasm. It is important to inform the patient that, while rare, sedation may occur, and therefore the author recommends that patients perform the trial over the weekend or during a period where they are not involved with high activity. For postmenopausal patients with vaginal dryness, compounding the medication into a vaginal suppository or coating it with a lubricant, such as coconut oil, may aid in liquification of the tablet.

7.3.5 Vestibular Cotton Swab Test (Q-Tip Test)

For patients with suspected vestibulodynia, the vestibular cotton swab test (Q-Tip test) is a way to confirm the anatomic location of their pain. The test is performed with the patient in the lithotomy position, with the labia minor gently separated to allow visualization of the vestibule. A cotton-tipped applicator is used to gently touch the vestibule in a clockwise fashion, and the patient is asked to describe if pain is present, as well as the quality of the pain.[182] Special attention should be paid to the periurethral (Skene's) glands, as well as the portion of the vestibule located above the urethra. A positive Q-Tip test is indicative of provoked vestibulodynia.

BOX 7.3

While not always present, there are associated "clock positions" with the different types of vestibulodynia. Pelvic floor–related pain is often present at 6 o'clock, while hormonal vestibulodynia tends to manifest in the upper half of the vestibule. Conversely, neuroproliferative vestibulodynia may be present throughout the entire vestibule, including the 12 o'clock position superior to the urethra.

7.3.6 Vestibular Anesthesia Test

Similar to the Q-Tip test, the vestibular anesthesia test (VAT) is a specialized testing modality to determine what degree of the patient's pain is related specifically to the vestibule. For the VAT, a cream made of topical anesthetic agents is applied to a large swab, and the mixture is painted over the vestibule. After approximately 15 minutes, a Q-Tip test is then performed to measure appropriate anesthesia of the tissue. Should the patient report significant improvement in their symptoms, the practitioner can assume that the vestibule is involved in the patient's condition.

BOX 7.4

The author uses a mixture of 20% benzocaine, 8% lidocaine, and 6% tetracaine, otherwise known as BLT cream, for their VAT, but other anesthetic mixes exist and can be equally effective.

7.3.7 Vulvar Dolorimetry

A dolorimeter is an instrument that is used to measure pain threshold and tolerance. Historically, it was first described in the 1940s by Hardy, Wolff, and Goodell, who used the heat of a focused 100-W projection lamp to increasingly heat study participants' skin until they felt pain, noting that most people expressed discomfort when their skin reached 113°F (45°C).[183] Since that initial experiment, multiple methods of determining pain sensitivities have been developed, with practical applications in many different realms of medicine. For sexual medicine practitioners, dolorimetry may be used to determine the exact amount of pressure needed for a patient to experience genital discomfort, but outside of the realm of research, it has little practical application. That said, if available, a vulvodolorimeter can be helpful in comparing differences in pain threshold based on laterality or to determine if neurologic compromise is present, although one could argue that a similar outcome could be determined by using previously discussed testing, such as the Q-Tip test or QST.

7.3.8 Vulvoscopy

As stated in Chapter 1, a vulvoscope is one of the most – if not the most – effective tools a sexual medicine provider has at their disposal. Vulvoscopy allows for magnified evaluation of the surface of the vulva, as well as for enhanced inspection of the clitoris, vestibule, and perineum. While there are a variety of different methods for performing vulvoscopy, the following protocol is one that is commonly used in sexual medicine practices (Figure 7.1).

1. Beginning at the mons pubis, the vulvoscope is turned to low magnification and an initial evaluation of the right labium magus is performed, progressing cephalad to caudad, with attention paid to the groin and hairline as well. This is carried down to the level of the perineum.
2. The perineum and perianal regions are then evaluated, and attention is turned to the posterior aspect of the patient's left labium magus.
3. The left labium magus is evaluated in a caudad-to-cephalad pattern, once again paying attention to the groin and hairline.
4. Once the mons pubis is reached, the left infralabial sulcus is then evaluated in a cephalad-to-caudad pattern until the posterior commissure of the vulva is reached.
5. This process is then repeated on the patient's right in a caudad-to-cephalad fashion, terminating at the anterior commissure.
6. The right labium minus is then evaluated cephalad to caudad, crossing the midline at the posterior fourchette, followed by caudad-to-cephalad evaluation of the left labium minus.
7. Magnification is increased, and the left clitoral frenulum, as well as the left aspect of the glans and hood of the clitoris, are then evaluated.
8. Proceeding in a cephalad-to-caudad fashion, the left vestibule is examined, with special attention paid to the Skene's and Bartholin's gland on that side. The midline is crossed at the posterior hymenal ring, and the right vestibule and accompanying structures are then evaluated caudad to cephalad, ending with evaluation of the right side of the clitoris.

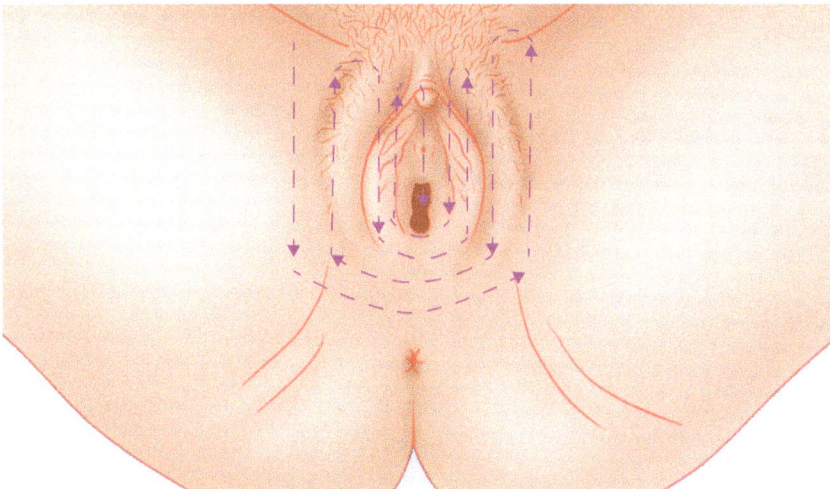

FIGURE 7.1   The technique of the vulvoscopy examination.

9. Finally, the midline structures of the vulva, including the urethra, are examined, with the vulvoscopy terminating with evaluation of the vaginal introitus.

By performing the vulvoscopy in this manner, the practitioner can be assured that they are evaluating the entirety of the vulva. For ease of documentation, a vulvoscopy template is available in Appendix 5.

7.4 Conclusion

The assessment of the female sexual medicine patient is complex and often involves a multifaceted approach utilizing a variety of different diagnostic modalities. Laboratory evaluation, focused imaging, and even sexual medicine–specific testing all have a place in the sexual medicine clinic and can aid the practitioner in finding, and treating, the appropriate dysfunction. Additionally, it is important to recognize that the field of sexual medicine is continuously evolving, with ongoing advancements in diagnostic technologies and treatment modalities appearing almost overnight in some cases. As such, it is imperative that clinicians remain abreast of the latest advances in the field, providing not only top-notch care but also the most accurate means of evaluating symptoms.

Despite these advances, however, it is important to not reduce patients to simply a list of lab results and radiologic impressions. Sexual medicine is, at its heart, a field concerned with connection – not simply the connection between one person to another but also between the provider and the patient. In order for patients to feel safe divulging their sexual fears and concerns, clinicians must provide a welcoming, respectful, and compassionate environment for the patient, one in which they feel that their provider actually cares about them and that they are, truly, not just a number.

7.5 Case Study

Theresa is a 34-year-old G3P3003 who presents complaining of worsening pain with intercourse. She states that over the past year she has noticed a burning, stinging pain along the superior aspect of her vestibule that has progressed to the point that penetration is now impossible. Additionally, she states that she cannot tolerate tampon insertion due to the discomfort. She denies any recent pelvic trauma but does admit to some exercise intolerance in her thighs. She has also recently had to visit the optometrist due to blurry vision. Which of the following testing modalities would be contraindicated in this patient?

A: Serum total testosterone level
B: Transvaginal sonography
C: Qualitive sensory nerve testing (QST)
D: MRI of brain with contrast

The answer is B. For patients with severe pain with penetration, transvaginal sonography is often not tolerated due to the discomfort that it may cause. Also, this patient has no findings that would suggest internal pelvic organ dysfunction as the cause of her concerns. None of the other testing modalities have contraindications and could all be utilized in the evaluation of this patient.

Chapter 8

Medical Therapies for Female Sexual Disorders

In the foreword to his book, *The Way of Qigong: The Art and Science of Chinese Energy Healing,* physician Larry Dossey wrote, "Modern medicine, as everyone knows by now, can be spectacularly successful and woefully inadequate. It alternately inspires praise and condemnation."[184] While Dr. Dossey's observations are more related to the differences between Western medical practice and Eastern philosophy, his opinion rings true when viewed through the lens of sexual medicine. Sexual medicine providers live in a world of constant juxtaposition, straddling the line between traditional, evidence-based practice and experimental innovation. As such, it is not uncommon for medications to be prescribed solely for off-label use or for interventions from other disciplines,

---

BOX 8.1

As discussed in Chapter 3, the concept of the biopsychosocial triad has been used to describe possible causes for a variety of different sexual concerns, and as such, it is only natural to use that same idea when discussing the different available treatment options for patients. As a guidebook primarily for sexual medicine practitioners, however, this chapter will focus mainly on the "biologic" aspect of that triad, deferring the psychological and/or sociologic sides of the triad for other publications.

DOI: 10.1201/9781003494522-8

TABLE 8.1 Quick Reference: Prescription Hormonal Medications

Hormone Therapy	Example Medication Names	Conditions Treated	Contraindications
Systemic Estradiol	Minivelle, Bijuva, Climara, Premarin, Femring, Depo-Estradiol	FSAD, PGAD/GPD, Vulvodynia, FOD	History of VTE, allergic reaction, AMI, CVA, estrogen-related cancer, known hypercoagulable disease, undiagnosed uterine bleeding
Vulvovaginal Estradiol	Estrace, Estring, Osphena, Premarin	FSAD, PGAD/GPD, Vulvodynia, FOD,	Undiagnosed uterine bleeding
Systemic Testosterone	Depo-Testosterone, AndroGel, Testim, Natesto,	HSDD, FSAD, FOD	Undiagnosed uterine/vaginal bleeding, pregnancy, allergic reaction, polycythemia, dyslipidemia
Vestibular Testosterone	Must be compounded	FSAD, PGAD/GPD, vulvodynia, FOD	Allergic reaction, pregnancy
Vaginal DHEA	Prasterone, Intrarosa	FSAD, PGAD/GPD, FOD	Undiagnosed uterine/vaginal bleeding, pregnancy
Oxytocin	Must be compounded	FOD	Pituitary tumor, Parkinson's disease

such as allergy and immunology, dermatology, or even aesthetics to be reverse-engineered for use in the sexual medicine world. It is paramount, therefore, that the sexual medicine provider understand not only the current therapies for sexual medicine conditions but also be ever vigilant for other possible treatment regimens, despite their source.

Current medical therapies for female sexual dysfunction can be separated into three distinct categories: prescription hormonal medication, prescription nonhormonal medication, and procedural/surgical treatments. The following sections will evaluate those types of therapies as they relate to the individual conditions noted in the previous chapters, with different preparations, associated conditions, mechanisms of action, dosages, and contraindications all described. For procedural/surgical treatments, a step-by-step guide will be provided to aid in appropriate techniques. Table 8.1 summarizes the therapies to be discussed.

8.1 Prescription Hormonal Medications
8.1.1 Systemic Estrogens

- Associated Condition(s): HSDD, FSAD, PGAD/GPD, Vulvodynia, FOD

TABLE 8.2 Systemic Estrogen Formulations and Dosages

Formulation	Dose Range and Frequency
Oral Tablet • Conjugated estrogens (equine) • Conjugated estrogens (synthetic) • Estradiol acetate • Micronized β estradiol (bioidentical)	0.35–2 mg daily
Transdermal • 17-β estradiol patch • 17-β estradiol gel • 17-β estradiol spray	0.025–0.1 mg daily/biweekly/weekly 1.53 mg estradiol per spray
Intravaginal Ring • Femring	0.05 mg, 0.01 mg every 3 months
Intramuscular • Estradiol cypionate • Estradiol valerate	1–5 mg monthly

8.1.1.1 Mechanism of Action

Systemic estrogen binds to either alpha or beta estrogen receptors (ERα and ERβ) located in various tissues throughout the body, including the reproductive organs, brain, bones, and cardiovascular system. Once bound, these receptors undergo conformational changes that trigger a downstream effect, such as the creation of neurotransmitters in the central nervous system, feedback control of the hypothalamic–pituitary–gonadal (HPG) axis, and regulation of the menstrual cycle. Table 8.2 lists the formulations and dosages.

8.1.1.2 Contraindications

- *Absolute*: Previous history of venous thromboembolism (VTE), allergic reaction, acute myocardial infarction (AMI), cerebrovascular accident (CVA), estrogen-related cancer, known hypercoagulable disease with history of VTE (factor V Leiden, prothrombin mutation, protein C or S deficiency), undiagnosed uterine/vaginal bleeding
- *Relative*: Increased risk of estrogen-related cancer, hypercholesterolemia, liver disease, renal disease, obesity, prolonged immobilization, angioedema, migraine with aura
- *Notes*: Mild effects in vulvovaginal tissue. More useful in treating menopause-related changes, such as vasomotor changes or catamenial anxiety or migraine. Femring provides both systemic and local estradiol replacement. Transdermal estradiol currently preferred over oral or injectable preparations due to better safety profile.[185] As estradiol is a steroid-based sex hormone, consider evaluation of cholesterol if using IM formulation. Patients who have a uterus must be on progestogen or tissue-selective estrogen blocking if using systemic estradiol.

TABLE 8.3 Vulvovaginal Estrogens and Associated Therapies

Formulation	Dose Range and Frequency
Oral Tablet • Ospemifene (SERM)	• 60 mg daily
Vaginal Cream • Conjugated estrogens (equine) • 17-β Estradiol	• 0.5–2 g (contains 0.0625 mg CEE/g) daily • 1 g (contains 0.1 mg 17-β estradiol) daily
Intravaginal Ring	2 mg (0.0075 mg estradiol daily)/3 months
Vaginal Suppository	4–25 mcg estradiol daily

8.1.2 Vulvovaginal Estrogens and Associated Therapies

- Associated Condition(s): Female sexual arousal disorder (FSAD), persistent genital arousal disorder/genitopelvic dysesthesia (PGAD/GPD), vulvodynia, female orgasm disorder (FOD), genitourinary syndrome of menopause (GSM), genitourinary syndrome of lactation (GSL)

8.1.2.1 Mechanism of Action

Binds to local estrogen receptors in vulvovaginal tissue. Aids with estrogenization of vulvovaginal mucosa. Increases vaginal lubrication. Increases number of superficial cells in vagina, which increases elasticity and trauma resistance. May increase genital sensitivity. Table 8.3 lists the therapies.

8.1.2.2 Contraindications

Undiagnosed uterine/vaginal bleeding, allergic reaction. Ospemifene has the same contraindications as systemic estrogen therapy.

8.1.2.3 Notes

No need for progestin therapy in patients who have a uterus if using vaginal estradiol therapy. Ospemifene *does* require progestogen or a tissue-selective estrogen blocker use to reduce risk of uterine cancer.

8.1.3 Systemic Testosterone

- Associated Condition(s): HSDD, FSAD, FOD

8.1.3.1 Mechanism of Action

Testosterone exerts its effects by binding to androgen receptors present in various tissues throughout the body, including the brain, muscles, and genitalia. Activation of androgen receptors leads to physiological changes such as promotion of neural circuits involved in sexual desire, motivation, mood, and cognitive function; genital effects such as clitoral sensitivity, vaginal lubrication, and tissue integrity; and increasing muscle strength and bone density. Table 8.4 lists the formulations.

BOX 8.2

There are no Food and Drug Administration (FDA)–approved formulations for testosterone replacement therapy in women. Therefore, it is current practice to dose systemic testosterone therapy at one-tenth the "male dose." As such, prescribers need to reduce the dosages listed in Table 8.4 to one-tenth of the dose when prescribing for a female patient.

TABLE 8.4 Systemic Testosterone Formulations

Formulation	Dose Range and Frequency (FOR MALE PATIENT)
Oral Tablets	
• Fluoxymesterone	• 5–20 mg daily
• Methyltestosterone	• 10–50 mg daily
Transdermal	
• Patch	• 2–6 mg daily
• Gel	• 10–120 mg daily
Transmucosal	
• Intransal	• 11 mg TID
• Buccal	• 30 mg BID
Intramuscular	
• Testosterone cypionate	• 150–200 mg biweekly
• Testosterone undecanoate	• 750 mg monthly × 2 months, then every 10 weeks

---

8.1.3.2 Contraindications

- *Absolute*: Undiagnosed uterine/vaginal bleeding, pregnancy, allergic reaction, polycythemia
- *Relative*: Dyslipidemia

8.1.3.3 Possible Alternatives

Due to the lack of FDA-approved testosterone therapy for women, many providers utilize compounding pharmacies for their ability to prepare appropriate doses for female patients. While these preparations may occur in many formulations, transdermal gels or creams are the most common form of compounded testosterone and are usually prescribed with a dose of 5–10 mg of testosterone daily.

8.1.3.4 Notes

Before initiating serum testosterone therapy, a serum complete blood count (CBC), liver function panel, lipid panel, and testosterone level should be drawn. Routine monitoring of testosterone levels is important to prevent side effects from the medication including hirsutism, alopecia, and acne, as well as preventing virilization effects such as voice deepening or clitoromegaly. There is not clear evidence to support lipid screening or liver function evaluation during treatment for transdermal testosterone outside of normal practices.[186]

8.1.4 Vestibular Testosterone

- Associated Condition(s): FSAD, PGAD/GPD, Vulvodynia, FOD

8.1.4.1 Mechanism of Action

Local hormone application binds to androgen receptors in vestibular epithelium and minor vestibular glands, decreasing inflammation and irritation and improving blood flow to the tissue. This in turn reduces pain and may improve lubrication.

8.1.4.2 Common Dosage

Vestibular testosterone must be compounded and is created at a lower dose than what is used with systemic therapy. Common dosages include 0.01% to 0.1% testosterone in a hypoallergic base.

8.1.4.3 Contraindications

- Allergic reaction, pregnancy

8.1.4.4 Notes

Very little systemic absorption. Not applicable for treatment of hypoandrogenism.

8.1.5 Vaginal Dehydroepiandrosterone (DHEA)

- Associated Condition(s): FSAD, PGAD/GPD, FOD

8.1.5.1 Mechanism of Action

As a prohormone, DHEA can be converted into both androgens and estrogens in various tissues of the body, including the vagina. This leads to stimulation of vaginal tissue and, more specifically, growth of vaginal epithelial cells, which increases the thickness of the vaginal lining. This can help improve vaginal lubrication and reduce symptoms of vaginal atrophy. In addition, vaginal androgen absorption can affect vestibular tissue, mimicking the effects of vestibular testosterone therapy.

8.1.5.2 Common Dosage

Vaginal DHEA therapy is commercially available in 6.5 mg suppositories that are inserted nightly into the vagina.

8.1.5.3 Contraindications

- Undiagnosed uterine/vaginal bleeding, allergic reaction, pregnancy

8.1.5.4 Notes

The suppository contains both coconut and palm oil, so caution is advised in patients with known sensitivities/allergies to those substances.

8.1.6 Oxytocin

- Associated Condition(s): FOD

8.1.6.1 Mechanism of Action

Oxytocin is thought to contribute to sexual activity and orgasm through several mechanisms including promoting feelings of relaxation and trust and increasing uterine contractions in females and contractions of the vas deferens and prostate in males, thereby theoretically intensifying orgasm, as well as interaction with dopamine and serotonin, both of which are involved in regulating mood, pleasure, and reward. Table 8.5 lists the formulations.

8.1.6.2 Contraindications

- *Absolute*: Pregnancy
- *Relative*: Hypertension, kidney disease

TABLE 8.5 Oxytocin Formulations

Formulation	Dose and Frequency
Intranasal	24–32 IU daily
Sublingual/Troche	50 IU daily or 1 hour prior to sexual activity

8.2 Nonhormonal Prescription Medications (Table 8.6)

TABLE 8.6 Quick Reference Table: Prescription Nonhormonal Medications

Medication Class	Example Medication Names	Conditions Treated	Contraindications
Serotonin agonist/ Antagonist	Flibanserin, Addyi	HSDD	Hypersensitivity/ allergy, excessive alcohol consumption, liver failure, pregnancy, breastfeeding
Selective Serotinin Reuptake Inhibitor (SSRI)/ Serotonin Norepinephrine Reuptake Inhibitor (SNRI)	Citalopram, escitalopram, paroxetine, duloxetine, venlafaxine, desvenlafaxine	Vulvodynia	Hypersensitivity/ allergy, MAO-I use within 14 days, liver disease, renal failure
Tricyclic Antidepressant (TCA)	Amitriptyline, nortriptyline	Vulvodynia	Hypersensitivity/ allergy, MAO-I use within 14 days, recent AMI
Norepinephrine-Dopamine Reuptake Inhibitor (NDRI)	Bupropion	HSDD	Hypersensitivity/ allergy, seizure disorder, MAO-I use within 14 days, anorexia/bulimia
CNS Stimulants	Methylphenidate, dextroamphetamine	HSDD	Hypersensitivity/ allergy, pregnancy, breastfeeding, MAO-I use within 14 days, CAD, cardiomegaly, GFR<15
Anticonvulsants	Gabapentin, pregabalin	Vulvodynia	Hypersensitivity/ allergy, creatinine clearance <30
PDE5 Inhibitor	Sildenafil, tadalafil	FSAD, FOD	Hypersensitivity/ allergy, nitrate use
Melanocortin Receptor Agonist	Bremelanotide, Vyleesi	HSDD	Hypersensitivity/ allergy, pregnancy, uncontrolled HTN, uncontrolled heart disease

(Continued)

TABLE 8.6 (Continued) Quick Reference Table: Prescription Nonhormonal
Medications

Medication Class	Example Medication Names	Conditions Treated	Contraindications
Botulinum Neurotoxin	OnabotulinumtoxinA, Botox	PFD, vulvodynia, vaginismus	Hypersensitivity/ allergy, albumin hypersensitivity
Local Anesthetics	Lidocaine, bupivacaine	Vulvodynia, vaginismus	Hypersensitivity/ allergy

8.2.1 Serotonin Agonist/Antagonist

- Associated Condition(s): HSDD, FSAD

8.2.1.1 Mechanism of Action

Not fully understood. Displays 5-HTA1 and 5-HTA2 receptor modulation, demonstrating agonist activity on 5-HTA1 receptors and antagonist activity on 5-HTA2 receptors, resulting in decreased levels of neuronal sexual inhibitory serotonin and increased dopamine and norepinephrine activity. Increased dopamine leads to increased sexual desire.

8.2.1.2 Common Dosage

- 100 mg PO at bedtime

8.2.1.3 Contraindications

- *Absolute*: Hypersensitivity/allergy, pregnancy, liver failure, excessive alcohol consumption
- *Relative*: Concomitant use of central nervous system (CNS) depressants, hypotension, syncope
- *Note*: If there is no change in symptoms after 8 weeks, discontinue medication. While FDA approved for premenopausal females, may be used off-label for postmenopausal patients

8.2.2 SSRI/SNRI

- Associated Condition(s): Vulvodynia

8.2.2.1 Mechanism of Action

SSRIs prevent the reuptake of serotonin in the brain, thereby increasing circulating amounts of the neurotransmitter. In addition to serotonin, SNRIs decrease norepinephrine absorption as well, which leads to a higher serum concentration of both transmitters, as well as increased noradrenaline in the synaptic cleft. This affects vulvodynia symptoms by inhibiting or decreasing neuropathic pain sensations.[187] Table 8.7 lists the formulations.

TABLE 8.7 Selective Serotonin Reuptake Inhibitor Formulations and Dosages

Medication	Dosage and Frequency (All Oral Formulations)
Paroxetine	10–20 mg daily
Duloxetine	60 mg daily
Citalopram	10–20 mg daily
Escitalopram	10–20 mg
Venlafaxine	75–225 mg ER daily

TABLE 8.8 Tricyclic Antidepressant Formulations and Dosages

Medication	Dosage and Frequency (All Oral Formulations)
Tertiary Amine Tricyclics	
• Amitriptyline	• 25–100 mg at bedtime
• Doxepin	• 2.5 mg/kg[189] at bedtime
• Imipramine	• 0.2–3 mg/kg at bedtime
Secondary Amine Tricyclics	
• Desipramine	• 100–150 mg daily (begin at 25 mg and taper)
• Nortriptyline	• 25–150 mg at bedtime (taper by 25 mg every 2–3 days)

8.2.2.2 Contraindications

Hypersensitivity/allergy, MAO-I use within 14 days, liver disease, renal failure.

8.2.2.3 Notes

Avoid abrupt discontinuation of medication. SSRIs are used mostly in conjunction with TCA or after failure of TCA.[188] Duloxetine has a separate indication for neuropathic pain.

8.2.3 Tricyclic Antidepressants (TCAs)

* Associated Condition(s): Vulvodynia

8.2.3.1 Mechanism of Action

TCAs function by blocking multiple neurotransmitter receptors, including serotonin, norepinephrine, and histamine, thereby decreasing nociceptor activity in both peripheral and spinal cord pain pathways. Tricyclics are divided into both tertiary and secondary amine subtypes, which have a greater inhibitory effect on serotonin or norepinephrine, respectively. Table 8.8 lists the formulations.

8.2.3.2 Contraindications

* *Absolute*: Allergy to TCA, recent myocardial infarction
* *Relative*: Glaucoma, thyroid disease, prostatic hypertrophy, urinary retention

8.2.3.3 Notes

Overall effective for neuropathic pain, but use is limited due to significant side effect profile including weight gain, orthostatic hypotension, dry mouth, and urinary retention. Accidental overdose has elevated risk of mortality.[190]

8.2.4 Norepinephrine-Dopamine Reuptake Inhibitor

- Associated Condition(s): HSDD

8.2.4.1 Mechanism of Action

Not fully understood. Inhibits reuptake of norepinephrine and dopamine, with dopamine uptake having a significantly higher degree of inhibition as compared to norepinephrine. May also have limited effect on nicotinic and serotonin receptors. Increased circulating dopamine is thought to increase sexual desire. Table 8.9 lists the formulations.

8.2.4.2 Contraindications

- *Absolute*: Allergy to NDRI, seizure disorders, history of anorexia or bulimia nervosa, current or recent use of monoamine oxidase inhibitors (MAO-Is), history of bipolar disorder
- *Relative*: Renal impairment, hepatic impairment, history of head trauma or brain injury, use of medications that lower the seizure threshold, high risk of suicide

8.2.4.3 Notes

The 150 mg dosage has been found to be more effective in treating hypoactive sexual desire disorder (HSDD) than the 300 mg dose.[191]

8.2.5 CNS Stimulants

- Associated Condition(s): HSDD

TABLE 8.9 Bupropion Formulation and Dosages

Medication	Dosage and Frequency (All Oral Formulations)
Bupropion SR	150 mg twice a day
Bupropion XL	150–300 mg every morning

TABLE 8.10 CNS Stimulant Formulations and Dosages

Medication	Dosage and Frequency (All Oral formulations)
Dextroamphetamine/Amphetamine	5–40 mg in divided doses
Dextroamphetamine	5–40 mg in divided doses
Methylphenidate IR Methylphenidate ER	10–60 mg daily 20–49 mg every morning
Lisdexamfetamine	30–70 mg every morning
Dexmethylphenidate Hydrochloride	2.5–10 mg twice a day

8.2.5.1 Mechanism of Action

CNS stimulants function by increasing serotonin, dopamine, and norepinephrine in the presynaptic cleft. They also weakly inhibit monoamine oxidase, which further increases the amount of dopamine available via reuptake inhibition. Table 8.10 lists the formulations.

8.2.5.2 Contraindications

- *Absolute*: Hypersensitivity or allergy, advanced arteriosclerosis, cardiovascular disease, moderate to severe hypertension, hyperthyroidism, glaucoma
- *Relative*: Symptomatic cardiovascular disease, seizure disorders, Tourette syndrome, history of motor or verbal tics, pregnancy, and breastfeeding

8.2.5.3 Notes

Limited use in patients without underlying attention/concentration disorder. On-demand use may decrease side effects but can lead to disordered sleep if taken too late in the day.

8.2.6 Anticonvulsants

- Associated Condition(s): Vulvodynia

8.2.6.1 Mechanism of Action

As a class, anticonvulsants modulate neuronal excitability and reduce hyperactivity in nociceptive gateways. They also decrease excitatory glutamate activity and amplify inhibition of neuronal activity by gamma-aminobutyric acid (GABA). This leads to a reduction in nerve conduction aberrancy, thereby decreasing neuropathic pain. Table 8.11 lists the formulations.

TABLE 8.11 Anticonvulsant Formulations and Dosages

Medication	Dosage and Frequency (All Oral Formulations)
Gabapentin	300–1200 mg every 8 hours
Pregabalin	50–100 mg every 8 hours
Lamotrigine	200–400 mg in divided doses

TABLE 8.12 PDE5 Inhibitor Formulations and Dosages

Medication	Dosage and Frequency (All Oral Formulations)
Sildenafil	20 mg given 0.5–1 hour prior to sexual activity
Tadalafil	2.5–5 mg daily

8.2.6.2 Contraindications

- *Absolute*: Hypersensitivity to the medication, severe liver disease, severe renal impairment
- *Relative*: Pregnancy and breastfeeding, respiratory depression, history of substance abuse, heart block or bradycardia, myasthenia gravis, chronic obstructive pulmonary disease (COPD)

8.2.6.3 Notes

Anticonvulsant medication dosage should be increased slowly to reduce medication-related side effects.

8.2.7 PDE5 Inhibitor

- Associated Condition(s): FSAD

8.2.7.1 Mechanism of Action

Inhibits phosphodiesterase 5 (PDE5), an enzyme which is responsible for disassembling cyclic guanosine monophosphate (cGMP) in smooth muscle cells, specifically in the genitalia. Sexual stimulation increases the production of nitric oxide, which in turn leads to elevation in cGMP and an influx of blood to the genitals. Inhibition of PDE5 therefore allows for increased genital vasodilation and an improvement in sexual arousal. Table 8.12 lists the formulations.

8.2.7.2 Contraindications

- *Absolute*: Use of nitrate medications (e.g., nitroglycerin), hypersensitivity to PDE5 inhibitors, severe hepatic impairment, severe renal impairment (creatinine clearance <30 mL/min)

- *Relative*: Uncontrolled hypertension, recent stroke or myocardial infarction, hereditary retinal disorders, unstable angina, sickle cell anemia

8.2.7.3 Notes

Common side effects include facial flushing and nasal congestion. Sildenafil may be compounded into a topical form and applied directly to the clitoris prior to sexual activity.

8.2.8 Melanocortin Receptor Agonist

- Associated Condition(s): HSDD, FSAD

8.2.8.1 Mechanism of Action

Melanocortin receptor agonists exert their mechanism of action by binding to hypothalamic melanocortin receptors. This binding increases the release of dopamine and competitively inhibits serotonin. The end effect is an increase in sexual excitation, thereby alleviating symptoms of HSDD.

8.2.8.2 Common Dosage

The dose is 1.75 mg injected SC at least 45 minutes prior to sexual activity.

8.2.8.3 Contraindications

- *Absolute*: Pregnancy, hypersensitivity to bremelanotide or any component of the formulation
- *Relative*: Uncontrolled hypertension, cardiovascular disease, history of cerebrovascular events, severe hepatic impairment, severe renal impairment

8.2.8.4 Notes

Common side effects include headache and nausea. Do not exceed more than one dose per 24-hour period. Although the typical duration of effect is 12 hours, some individuals may experience significantly longer periods of effect.

8.2.9 Botulinum Neurotoxin

- Associated Condition(s): Vulvodynia, vaginismus, PFD

8.2.9.1 Mechanism of Action

Neurotoxins exert their therapeutic effects by inhibiting the release of acetylcholine at the neuromuscular junction. This effect leads to weakened or blocked muscular contraction, which may provide relief for conditions associated with muscle spasm.

8.2.9.2 Common Dosage

Botulinum neurotoxins are prepacked as a powder, usually in 100-unit bottles, and require reconstitution with sterile saline prior to injection. The total amount injected, as well as the ratio of botulinum toxin to saline, is variable dependent on the size of the muscle being injected, as well as the desired spread.

8.2.9.3 Contraindications

- *Absolute*: Known hypersensitivity to botulinum toxin, presence of infection at the proposed injection site(s), myasthenia gravis, or Lambert-Eaton syndrome
- *Relative*: Pregnancy or breastfeeding, neuromuscular disorders other than myasthenia gravis or Lambert-Eaton syndrome, concurrent use of aminoglycosides or other agents interfering with neuromuscular transmission

8.2.9.4 Notes

The various formulations of botulinum toxins have different onsets of action, as well as duration of effects. Additionally, as botulinum is a paralytic agent, care needs to be taken when injecting near muscular sphincters, such as the anus or urethra, to avoid possible unintentional incontinence as a side effect of injection.

8.2.10 Local Anesthetic

- Associated Condition(s): Vulvodynia, vaginismus

8.2.10.1 Mechanism of Action

The mechanism of action for local anesthetics involve blocking sodium channels along nerves. This inhibition of sodium ion activity effectively decreases the generation of nerve action potentials, thereby preventing pain signaling from traveling to the brain from the affected tissue. Table 8.13 lists the formulations.

8.2.10.2 Contraindications

Known allergy or sensitivity to local anesthetic.

8.2.10.3 Notes

Topical formulations of both lidocaine and bupivacaine are available and may be applied prior to sexual activity to help decrease pain with penetration.

TABLE 8.13 Local Anesthetic Agent Formulations and Dosages

Medication	Dosage and Frequency (All Injected)
Lidocaine	0.5–1% solution, usually 1–5 mL per injection site
Bupivacaine	0.25–0.5% solution, typically 1–2 mL per injection site
Marcaine (bupivacaine and epinephrine)	0.25–0.5% solution, usually 1–2 mL per injection site

Avoid injection of epinephrine-containing local anesthetics into the clitoris. Lidocaine has a more rapid onset but relatively short duration. Bupivacaine has longer onset time but has longer-lasting effects.

BOX 8.3 LUBRICANTS AND MOISTURIZERS

There are a plethora of commercially available vaginal lubricants and moistures that are often marketed to women who experience vaginal dryness or who simply wish to increase lubrication during sexual activity. Although the terms lubricant and moisturizer are colloquially interchangeable, they are vastly different substances in the sexual medicine world. Lubricants are to be used during sexual activity and help amplify, or replace, the natural vaginal transudate produced with sexual activity. Moisturizers, on the other hand, are to be used irrespective of sexual activity and create a barrier along the mucosa of the vagina as a means to combat vaginal dryness outside of sex.

Vaginal lubricants come in three different base formulations – water, oil, and silicone – each of which has a different set of characteristics that the sexual medicine provider should understand. Water-based lubricants are found with or without glycerin, are relatively short lasting, and may need to be reapplied during prolonged sexual activity. They are safe to use with condoms and arousal tools, however, and considered safe to use with oral sex. Oil-based lubricants are derived from natural oils such as olive or coconut oil and often provide a moisturizing effect as well as acting as a lubricant. They may affect vaginal pH, however, and can also decrease the efficacy of condoms. Oil-based lubricants, unless specifically noted, are not safe to use with arousal tools. Silicone-based lubricants typically last the longest of any lubricant and are generally considered hypoallergic and are therefore good for patients with sensitive skin. They are mostly safe for condom and arousal tool usage but may be messy to clean up.

Similarly, vaginal moisturizers are often water, oil, or silicone derived but have different properties that work better outside of sexual activity. Additionally, some moisturizers are considered safe for the vulva as well and therefore can serve a double purpose for patients with vulvovaginal dryness. Finally, some moisturizers include hyaluronic acid, a very potent moisturizing agent that has been studied as a viable alternative to vaginal estrogens in patients who are not candidates for vaginal hormone therapy.

TABLE 8.14 Quick Reference: Surgical and Procedural Interventions

Name of Procedure	Correlated Sexual Medicine Conditions
Trigger point injection	Vulvodynia, PFD
Pelvic floor chemodenervation	PFD, vaginismus, vulvodynia
Genital nerve block	Vulvodynia, PFD, PGAD/GPD
Clitoral debridement	Clitorodynia, PGAD/GPD, FOD
Lysis of clitoral adhesions	Clitorodynia, PGAD/GPD, FOD
Dorsal slit procedure	Clitorodynia, PGAD/GPD, FOD
Perineoplasty	Vulvodynia, dyspareunia
Vestibulectomy	Vestibulodynia

8.3 Surgical and Procedural Interventions (Table 8.14)

8.3.1 Trigger Point Injection

- *Introduction*: First described by Dr. Janet Travell in 1943, trigger points are localized "knots" of tightened muscle that cause pain. Associated with both acute and repetitive trauma, trigger points often present as palpable areas of tissue turgor and are associated with both focal and referred pain. The purpose of a trigger point injection is to create a temporary relaxation of the muscle, thereby increasing vascular perfusion, lengthening muscle fibers, and clearing inflammatory metabolites from the muscle.
- *Indication*: Myofascial Trigger Point(s)
- *Anesthesia required*: None
- *Procedure in detail*: Prior to the procedure, the desired local anesthetic agent is drawn into a syringe and a 25G needle is attached. Once a trigger point is identified, the area is locally cleaned with an appropriate cleaning solution. The needle is then injected at a 30-degree angle until the trigger point is reached. Aspiration is then performed to assure an avascular location. A small amount of the local anesthetic is then injected, and the needle is then slightly withdrawn but

without fully withdrawing from the muscle. The angle of the needle is then slightly changed, and the process repeated as many times as necessary to eliminate pain along the trigger point. The needle is then fully withdrawn, and a dressing is applied if needed. If additional trigger points are identified, the process may then be repeated.

- *Possible complications*: Pain, bleeding, infection, vascular injury, hematoma
- *Postoperative instructions*: Avoid strenuous activity to the injected muscle(s) for the next 24 hours
- *Notes*: To access pelvic floor muscles, a transvaginal approach is often used. A speculum should be placed to facilitate visualization of the injection site, and a pelvic floor exam needs to be performed prior to the injection to correctly identify trigger points.

8.3.2 Pelvic Floor Chemodenervation

- *Introduction*: Pelvic floor chemodenervation involves injecting botulinum neurotoxins into spasmed pelvic floor muscles to aid in relaxation. While the procedure can, and is often, performed on its own, it also works extremely well as an adjunct intervention to pelvic floor physical therapy. Due to the local spread of the botulinum toxin, multiple injections are often used to achieve a successful denervation, and, unlike with cosmetic botulinum injection, it is not uncommon to use 100 or 200 units of botulinum toxin to achieve results.
- *Indication*: Pelvic Floor Dysfunction (High-Tone)
- *Anesthesia required*: None required, although many practitioners will provide preoperative anxiolytics or nitrous oxide, or even perform the procedure under monitored anesthesia care (MAC) to facilitate patient relaxation.
- *Procedure in detail*: Prior to the procedure, the desired amount and concentration of the botulinum toxin mixture is prepared and drawn into a syringe, and a 27G needle is attached. If applicable, anesthesia is initiated and the area(s) of injection identified and appropriately cleaned. If necessary, a speculum may be inserted to aid with visualization of the deeper pelvic floor. The botulinum toxin mixture is then injected into the muscle belly using a "peppering technique," wherein multiple injections are made, with each one delivering a small amount of botulinum toxin mixture. This is done to fully ensure that the muscle belly receives as much mixture as possible. If multiple muscle groups are affected, the process is then repeated in each muscle. The needle is then fully removed and a dressing is applied if needed.
- *Possible complications*: Pain, infection at injection site(s), urinary or fecal incontinence

- *Postoperative instructions*: Avoid strenuous activity for the next 48 hours. Avoid sexual activity for 48 hours. Tylenol or ibuprofen may be used to aid with injection site discomfort.
- *Notes*: It takes approximately 72 hours for the injection to begin to take effect. As such, it is important to establish appropriate expectations for the patient prior to the procedure. They may resume pelvic floor therapy one week after the procedure. On average, patients may expect approximately 90 days' worth of effect from the botulinum toxin.

8.3.3 Genital Nerve Block

- *Introduction*: Genital nerve blocks are tools that can be used for both diagnostic and therapeutic indications. By eliminating, or at least greatly decreasing, genital nerve pain, the savvy practitioner can determine the extent of nerve involvement in their patient's complaint. Genital nerve blocks are divided into *pudendal, perineal, and dorsal clitoral* varieties, and while the exact location of the nerve blockade may be different, the procedure for the block is basically the same. In addition, a genital nerve block may be performed prior to another sexual medicine procedure to help aid with procedural pain control.
- *Indication*: Genital Pain
- *Anesthesia required*: None required, although many practitioners will provide preoperative anxiolytics or nitrous oxide, or even perform the procedure under MAC to facilitate patient relaxation.
- *Procedure in detail*: Prior to the procedure, the desired local anesthetic agent is drawn into a syringe and a needle is attached. The length and gauge of the needle are dependent on the site of the block, with a pudendal block requiring the longest and largest bore needle (often a 23G spinal needle), while a clitoral nerve block only requires a 0.5-inch, 30G needle. The desired injection site is identified and cleaned in standard fashion.

8.3.3.1 Pudendal Block

The patient is placed in dorsal lithotomy position, and a gloved index finger is inserted into the vagina. The ischial spine is then identified by palpation along the posterolateral vaginal sidewalls. If the ischial spines cannot be palpated directly, the sacrospinous ligament should be identified by palpating from the sacrum to the respective ischial spine. A needle guide, such as an Iowa Trumpet, or a trimmed spinal needle guard, is introduced and placed against the vaginal mucosa along the sacrospinous ligament, located approximately 1 cm inferomedial to the ischial spine. The needle is then inserted into the guide, and the ligament is punctured until a loss of resistance is noted. Avascular placement is confirmed, and the local anesthetic is injected. If necessary, the process may be repeated on the contralateral side. All instruments are then removed, and the patient is assessed for pain relief.

8.3.3.2 Perineal Block

The patient is placed in dorsal lithotomy position, and the perineum identified. A syringe containing local anesthesia is brought to the procedural field and a 27G needle is attached. The practitioner's nondominant thumb is placed directly medial to the ischial tuberosity, and the perineum is then injected in a semilunar pattern, with the nondominant thumb moving medial to the contralateral ischial tuberosity once the perineal midline is reached. Pinprick test is then performed to confirm anesthesia.

8.3.3.3 Dorsal Clitoral Nerve Block

The patient is placed in the dorsal lithotomy position and the clitoris identified. A syringe containing local anesthetic with a 30G needle attached is brought to the procedural field. The dorsal clitoral nerve location is identified by imagining a clockface overlying the clitoris and identifying the 2 o'clock and 10 o'clock positions. Approximately 5 mL of local anesthetic is injected approximately 2 cm laterally and 1 cm cephalad from the corpus of the clitoris. This process is then repeated on the contralateral side. The patient is then assessed for appropriate pain control.

- *Possible complications*: Injection site pain, injection site infection, neurovascular injury (rare)
- *Postoperative instructions*: Routine postinjection care
- *Notes*: Depending on the type of local anesthetic used, pain relief may occur almost immediately or take upwards of 30 minutes to become effective. Additionally, the duration of the effects from the nerve block can vary greatly, lasting from minutes to months, depending on the patient.

8.3.4 Clitoral Debridement

- *Introduction*: Despite adequate hygiene, many patients who present with clitoral pain are found upon examination to have a significant amount of debris underneath the clitoral hood. This debris may include pubic hair, sebaceous material, dirt, or more. The most bothersome type of clitoral debris are collections of desquamated epithelia cells that mix with smegmatic discharge to form what are known as "keratin pearls." The presence of keratin pearls underneath the clitoral hood often evokes a sensation patients describe as being not unsimilar to the feeling of an entrapped grain of sand or eyelash in the eye. This procedure, therefore, is aimed at cleaning out the accumulated material, including keratin pearls, underneath the clitoral hood as a means to alleviate patient discomfort.

- *Indication*: Clitoral Pain, Significant Debris, Presence of Keratin Pearls
- *Anesthesia required*: Due to the sensitivity of the clitoris, it is recommended to, at a minimum, apply a topical numbing cream to the tissue. If a numbing cream is not available, consider dorsal clitoral nerve block, pudendal block, or MAC.
- *Procedure in detail*: The patient is placed in the dorsal lithotomy position, and the glans of the clitoris is identified. Anesthetic cream is applied, and a dorsal clitoral nerve block is performed. Once anesthesia is confirmed, the hood of the clitoris is retracted to achieve visualization of the clitoral glans, with the goal of visualizing the corona. At this point, a small rigid dilator, such as a lacrimal duct dilator, is used to sweep away any loose debris. Any remaining debris, including keratin pearls, are individually removed using a mosquito forceps or other atraumatic tissue forceps. The clitoris is then irrigated to remove any residue. If necessary, lysis of clitoral adhesions may be performed during this procedure as well. The patient is then taken out of lithotomy position, and postprocedure care is discussed.
- *Possible complications*: Pain, infection, neurovascular damage
- *Postoperative instructions*: Apply ice to the clitoris as needed for the next 24 hours. Most patients are able to control pain with over-the-counter (OTC) pain medication, such as acetaminophen or ibuprofen.
- *Notes*: As some keratin pearls can be extremely small, the author performs this procedure under magnification using surgical loupes. If being performed in the operating room with other procedures, an operative microscope can also be used if the surgeon is familiar with usage. In the office setting, the magnification from a vulvoscope is often adequate to visualize small keratin pearls.

8.3.5 Lysis of Clitoral Adhesions

- *Introduction*: Often occurring in conjunction with clitoral debris, clitoral adhesions are filmy bands of connective tissue that form between the prepuce and the glans of the clitoris. These adhesions are usually due to an underlying inflammation or balanitis of the glans and may be severe enough to cause a phimosis of the clitoral hood. Clitoral adhesions are found in approximately 22% of patients seeking care for sexual dysfunction[192] and yet are often overlooked as a symptom of sexual pain. Much like clitoral hood debridement, the purpose of this procedure is to remove adhesions, thereby decreasing clitoral pain.

- *Indication*: Clitoral Pain, Clitoral Phimosis
- *Anesthesia required*: Due to the sensitivity of the clitoris, it is recommended to, at a minimum, apply a topical numbing cream to the tissue. If a numbing cream is not available, consider dorsal clitoral nerve block, pudendal block, or MAC.
- *Procedure in detail*: The patient is placed in the dorsal lithotomy position, and the glans of the clitoris is identified. Anesthetic cream is applied, and a dorsal clitoral nerve block is performed. Once anesthesia is confirmed, the hood of the clitoris is retracted to achieve visualization of the clitoral glans, with the goal of visualizing the corona. If a clitoral phimosis is identified, its severity should be noted in the patient's chart. A 4 × 4 gauze pad is then brought onto the procedure field, and the clitoral hood is bluntly dissected off the glans. If necessary, mosquito forceps or a lacrimal duct probe can be used to further lyse adhesions. A clitoral hood debridement may be performed during this procedure as well. An emollient is then applied to the newly released clitoral hood. The patient is taken out of lithotomy position, and postprocedure care is discussed.
- *Possible complications*: Pain, Infection, Neurovascular Injury
- *Postoperative instructions*: Apply ice to the clitoris as needed for the next 24 hours. Most patients are able to control pain with OTC medication, such as acetaminophen or ibuprofen. For the next week the patient is instructed to gently retract the clitoral hood daily and to apply an emollient to prevent recurrence of adhesions.
- *Notes*: As with clitoral hood debridement, magnification is extremely helpful in performing this procedure.

8.3.6 Dorsal Slit Procedure

- *Introduction*: In cases of moderate-to-severe clitoral phimosis, a nonsurgical lysis of the clitoral hood is often not effective in fully reducing symptoms. In these cases, the dorsal slit procedure may be used to aid in treating the underlying phimosis. While most often used in patients with lichen sclerosus or severe GSM, the dorsal slit procedure can be performed on any patient with moderate or severe clitoral phimosis and, if performed correctly, has a very high rate of success in treating recalcitrant clitoral adhesions.[193]
- *Indication*: Moderate-to-Severe Clitoral Phimosis

- *Anesthesia required*: Dorsal slit procedures are performed under general anesthesia or monitored anesthesia care and in conjunction with a dorsal clitoral nerve block.
- *Procedure in detail*: The patient is placed in dorsal lithotomy position, and the genitals are prepped and draped in sterile fashion. A dorsal clitoral nerve block is performed to aid in postoperative pain control. A lacrimal duct probe is inserted underneath the adhered clitoral hood, and a plane is established between the glans and prepuce. A mosquito forceps is inserted cephalad along the midline, and the skin of the prepuce is crushed in the forceps, creating a "crush line." Iris scissors are then used to create an incision along the crush line until the superior aspect of the glans, up to the corona, is visualized. The newly created flaps of the prepuce are then trimmed. As this incision will separate the outer and inner layers of the prepuce, dissolvable sutures are placed to reconnect those tissue layers, with the apex of the incision and the lateral borders of the slit being common sites. After hemostasis is obtained, an emollient is applied to the surgical site.
- *Possible complications*: Pain, infection, bleeding, neurovascular damage, increased clitoral sensitivity
- *Postoperative instructions*: Apply ice to the clitoris as needed for the next 24 hours. Most patients are able to control pain with OTC medication, such as acetaminophen or ibuprofen. For the next week the patient is instructed to gently retract the clitoral hood daily and to apply an emollient to prevent recurrence of adhesions. Sitz baths may be started 72 hours postoperatively if desired.
- *Notes*: Due to the possibility of increased clitoral sensitivity with this procedure, care must be taken to not remove too much of the clitoral hood, thereby exposing the clitoral body behind the corona. The author routinely uses 4-0 chromic gut suture for this procedure, but other types of sutures may be used as desired.

8.3.7 Perineoplasty

- *Introduction*: While a perineoplasty is often considered part of a posterior colporrhaphy, there are times in which a patient may be a candidate for this specific procedure outside of pelvic floor reconstruction. Common indications for perineoplasties include extensive scar tissue along the perineum secondary to trauma, poorly healed obstetric lacerations, or perineum-focused defects. The term perineoplasty is often used synonymously with perineorrhaphy, although the latter technically refers to the suturing, or tightening, of the perineum and introitus and is used more in a cosmetic sense as opposed to a reconstructive one.

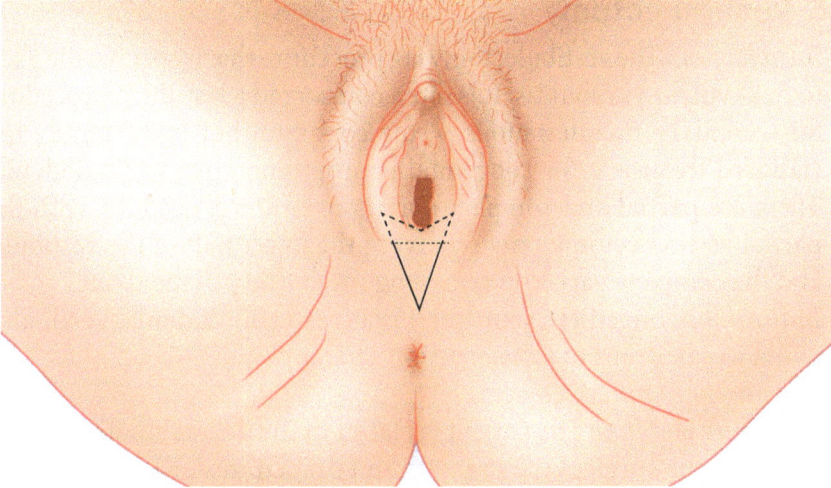

FIGURE 8.1   The final marking.

- *Indication*: Dyspareunia, Vulvodynia, PFD
- *Anesthesia required*: General
- *Procedure in detail*: The patient is placed in dorsal lithotomy position and the vulva and vagina are prepped and draped in sterile fashion. A surgical marking pen is used to create a "V" along the perineum, with the apex ending below the level of the defect and the arms of the V reaching the introitus. The marking pen is then used to extend the arms of the V into the vagina, and a shallow V is created past the level of the vestibule (Figure 8.1).

  - The area underneath the marking is then injected with local anesthetic. A 15-blade scalpel is then used to excise the marked tissue, including the underlying scar tissue. Once all of the scar tissue has been removed, the underlying dead space is reapproximated, and a vaginal free flap is then created by dissecting the vaginal mucosa off the rectovaginal fascia from the apex of the vaginal V and pulling it forward to the level of the introitus. It is then sutured in a tension-free fashion using dissolvable mattress stiches. The remaining vaginal aspects of the incision are then closed using interrupted sutures, and the perineal skin incision is then closed in a subcuticular fashion.

- *Possible complications*: Pain, infection, hematoma formation
- *Postoperative instructions*: Apply ice as needed for the next 24 hours. No tub soaks or swimming for four weeks, although sitz baths may be used after 72 hours. No sexual activity for four weeks. Avoid strenuous activity or exercise for four weeks.
- *Notes*: Postdelivery "peri-care" instructions can be substituted for this procedure, as it is very similar in terms of healing to a repaired obstetric laceration.

8.3.8 Vestibulectomy

- *Introduction*: The vestibulectomy is a procedure that is specifically used to treat vulvar vestibulitis. It is often considered a last-ditch procedure for secondary manifestations of the condition but is conversely the standard treatment for congenital neuroproliferative vestibulodynia. There are partial and complete variations of the procedure, with the partial vestibulectomy only removing the lower half of the vestibule, and the complete variation removing the entirety of the tissue.
- *Indication*: Congenital Neuroproliferative Vestibulodynia, Vestibulodynia Recalcitrant to Conservation Therapy
- *Anesthesia required*: General
- *Procedure in detail*: The patient is placed in the dorsal lithotomy position, and the surgical site prepped and draped in sterile fashion. The labia minora are retracted laterally to allow complete visualization of the vestibule. The intended incisional area is outlined with a surgical marking pen, beginning 1 mm laterally to the urethral meatus and proceeding superiorly for several centimeters before passing laterally to Hart's line and finally roughly 2 cm below the posterior fourchette. If the patient has pain at the 12 o'clock position in the tissue superior to the urethra, that tissue can be marked as well. Local anesthesia is then injected in the marked area not only for pain control but also to aid with hydrodissection. The marked area is then removed en bloc, at a depth of approximately 3 mm. This may be sent to pathology for confirmation of neuroproliferation if desired.[194]

  - Reconstruction of the tissue begins by closing the anterior and lateral dead space with dissolvable interrupted sutures. The posterior aspect of the excision is then repaired by creating a vaginal free flap by dissecting the vaginal tissue off the rectovaginal fascia. This flap is then sutured in a tension-free fashion, bringing the posterior vagina to the introitus. Additional local anesthetic can be injected if desired, or a pudendal block can be performed for more complete pain control.

- *Possible complications*: Pain, infection, hematoma, neurovascular damage, urinary retention
- *Postoperative instructions*: Apply ice as needed for the next 24 hours. No tub soaks or swimming for four weeks, although sitz baths may be used after 72 hours. Begin dilator therapy/physical therapy at four weeks. No sexual activity for six weeks. Avoid strenuous activity or exercise for six weeks.
- *Notes*: Due to the anatomic location of the Bartholin glands, patients who undergo vestibulectomy have an increased likelihood of developing Bartholin gland cysts or abscesses, as the ostia of the glands may be compromised as part of the surgery or in the healing process.[195]

8.4 Conclusion

It is an all-too-common occurrence for patients to present to the sexual medicine clinic frustrated by the lack of treatment options for their concerns. At the time of this writing, there are two FDA-approved medications for low sex drive in women (and only premenopausal women at that) and no formulations of testosterone, even though the ovaries make as much, if not more, testosterone on a daily basis than they make estrogens![196] Compare this to the number of medications for male sexual dysfunction, and it is no surprise that many providers feel hampered by the lack of possible treatment options for their patients. While psychotherapy and physiotherapy undoubtably have a place in helping patients with sexual concerns, the sexual medicine provider must also be comfortable with the current medications – FDA approved or otherwise – that may benefit their patients. Additionally, a thorough knowledge of available, and safe, hormone therapies is required, as so many sexual conditions have hormonal components. Finally, although not all sexual medicine providers are proceduralists, it is still important to at least have a basic understanding of what specialized procedures are available for patients, as discussions about surgical or procedural intervention will undoubtably arise.

8.5 Case Study

Daria is a 57-year-old menopausal female who presents with a history of worsening vulvar pain. She states that the pain is most prevalent with sitting, although sexual penetration seems to make it worse. She denies any chronic medical conditions, stating that she is "really healthy," admitting to riding her bike at least 10 miles a day. She does not take any medications, nor has she been on hormone therapy. She states that the pain is burning in quality and radiates up to the clitoris. Upon examination you find right-sided hyperalgesia along the labium magus and clitoris, as well as pain extending to the midline of the perineum. She also exhibits signs of vaginal dryness and loss of vulvar architecture. Which of the following treatment options are appropriate for this patient?

 A: Pudendal nerve block
 B: Gabapentin 300 mg TID
 C: 17-β Estradiol vaginal cream
 D: All of the above

The answer is D. This patient has a presentation that is highly suspicious for pudendal neuralgia, and as such, a pudendal nerve block is an appropriate diagnostic, and possibly therapeutic, option for therapy. In addition, gabapentin is a standard medication for vulvodynia, and the 300 mg dose three times a day is an appropriate starting dosage. Finally, as the patient is menopausal and demonstrates signs of genitourinary changes related to menopause, the addition of vaginal estradiol cream would be indicated.

Chapter **9**

Sexual Function Metrics and Questionnaires

Sexual function metrics exist to apply quantitative measurements to symptoms or behavior that is often qualitative in nature. Outside of general measurements of bodily function – blood pressure and the like – it is simply not possible to evaluate changes in sexual function in terms of millimeters, deciliters, or pounds per square inch. As such, specific metrics have been created to aid in the evaluation of both sexual function and dysfunction, as well as the changes that occur in patients who present with sexual concerns.

As a whole, sexual function metrics are more suited to the realms of research than to actual clinical practice. Many patients are resistant to filling out surveys prior to every visit, and most electronic medical records do not have sexual medicine questionnaires built into their software. That said, as most sexual medicine research utilizes at least one of the following scales, the ability to interpret the results of the different questionnaires is invaluable to accurately understand study data. Finally, while it is obviously important to understand what each metric is used for, it is equally important to keep in mind that the metrics do have limitations in their use.

As such, this chapter will divide the metrics into five distinct parts: development and validation, structure and content, administration and use, application and implications, and strengths and limitations. Measurements of statistical strength, such as test-retest reliability, Cronbach's alpha, and

DOI: 10.1201/9781003494522-9

the like, will be included if available. Additionally, as this chapter is meant to highlight practical applications of the metrics, an in-depth analysis of every metric available is beyond the scope of this publication. Curious readers should instead follow the endnotes provided to view the source material of the individual metrics or seek the aid of a medical librarian to find identify specific articles. Finally, not every domain of female sexual dysfunction has a separate, specific metric. As such, should a questionnaire for a domain not covered in this chapter be needed, the author recommends using one of the scales for assessing multiple domains of sexual dysfunction.

9.1 Scales for Assessment of Multiple Domains of Sexual Dysfunction

9.1.1 Sexual Function Questionnaire

The Sexual Function Questionnaire (SFQ)[197] is a 34-item questionnaire specifically designed to assess sexual function in female participants. It evaluates seven domains of sexual functioning, including two subtypes of sexual arousal. A shorter version of the SFQ titled the SFQ-28 is also available.[198]

9.1.1.1 Development and Validation

The SFQ was developed to provide a way to assess measures of sexual health in a reliable and comprehensive fashion. Since its origin, it has been validated through numerous studies and demonstrates an internal consistency value of 0.65 to 0.91 as well as high test-retest reliability, with a Cohen's weighted kappa of 0.21 to 0.71 and a Pearson's correlation coefficient of 0.42 to 0.78. Its Cronbach's α is 0.70 to 0.93 for subjects with female sexual arousal disorder (FSAD) and hypoactive sexual desire disorder (HSDD), respectively.

9.1.1.2 Structure and Content

The SFQ evaluates sexual desire, physical arousal-sensation, physical arousal-lubrication, enjoyment, orgasm, pain, and partner relationship. The scoring system aggregates responses into specific subscale scores as well as a total score, allowing for ease with interpretation.

9.1.1.3 Administration and Use

The questionnaire is designed for adult participants and can be completed by the patient or administered by the clinician. It has been adapted for various demographic groups and is flexible enough to be used in both clinic and research settings.

9.1.1.4 Applications and Implications

From a clinical standpoint, the SFQ helps in quantifying sexual dysfunction as well as guiding treatment plans. In research, it serves as a tool for identifying sexual health trends, monitoring treatment outcomes, and assessing the impact of interventions on sexual function.

9.1.1.5 Strengths and Limitations

The SFQ provides a general overview of female sexual function and is one of the better metrics for evaluating FSAD specifically. That said, it was mainly developed to assess for dysfunction related to specific comorbidities or drug-related sexual function and therefore may not be applicable for all patients.

9.1.2 Female Sexual Function Index

The Female Sexual Function Index (FSFI)[199] is a specialized, multidimensional metric developed to evaluate sexual function in female participants. It is extensively used in both clinical and research settings.

9.1.2.1 Development and Validation

The FSFI was created to assess female-specific sexual concerns and provide a similar metric to those already available for male patients. It has been validated in multiple follow-up studies and is often considered the primary metric for generalized female sexual dysfunction. It has high statistical strength, reporting test-retest reliability of 0.79 to 0.86 for each domain, as well as a Cronbach's α of 0.82 and higher.

9.1.2.2 Structure and Content

The FSFI evaluates patient experiences over the past 30 days in terms of six domains: desire, arousal, lubrication, orgasm, satisfaction, and pain. Each domain includes specific questions that participants rate, which are then aggregated into domain scores as well as an overall score.

9.1.2.3 Administration and Use

The FSFI is intended for use with adult females experiencing sexual concerns. It is typically given as a self-reported questionnaire, although it may be administered by clinicians or research personnel. The test itself is readily available online and contains clear guidelines, which ensure consistent administration and scoring.

9.1.2.4 Applications and Implications

Clinically, the FSFI is helpful in diagnosing various sexual dysfunctions, as well as tracking the progress of dysfunction-related interventions. In the research setting, it is widely used to evaluate the impact of various therapies on female sexual health as well as to explore sexual function and dysfunction trends across different populations.

9.1.2.5 Strengths and Limitations

The FSFI's main strength is its comprehensive evaluation of female sexual function, allowing it to be used in a variety of settings. However, limitations include potential cultural biases, the challenges inherent in self-reporting, and a retrospective time frame of only 30 days, which may render it useless for patients who are not currently sexually active.

9.2 Scales for Assessment of Sexual Desire

9.2.1 Decreased Sexual Desire Screener

The Decreased Sexual Desire Screener (DSDS)[200] is a brief diagnostic tool designed to identify HSDD in female participants. It is used primarily in clinical settings to quickly assess whether a patient's low sexual desire may be due to HSDD.

9.2.1.1 Development and Validation

The DSDS was developed to provide a quick and effective screening method for HSDD for clinicians who do not specialize in sexual medicine. The DSDS was found to have a sensitivity and specificity of 83.6% and 87.8%, respectively, for allowing nonspecialized clinicians to diagnose HSDD.

9.2.1.2 Structure and Content

The DSDS consists of five questions that focus on various aspects of sexual desire as well as its impact on personal distress. This format allows for rapid administration and scoring, aiding with the real-time diagnosis of HSDD.

9.2.1.3 Administration and Use

The DSDS is targeted at adult female patients experiencing low sexual desire. It can be self-administered or conducted by a clinician during a routine office visit.

9.2.1.4 Applications and Implications

Clinically, the DSDS is used to screen for HSDD, allowing clinicians to decide whether further evaluation or treatment is necessary. As a side note, it may also facilitate discussions about sexual health between patients and healthcare providers, which can aid in better patient outcomes.

9.2.1.5 Strengths and Limitations

The DSDS is valued for its brevity and ease of use, making it a practical tool in clinical environments. It is limited to HSDD, however, which decreases its efficacy in evaluating other causes of low sexual desire.

9.2.2 Sexual Desire Inventory

The Sexual Desire Inventory (SDI)[201] is a comprehensive, self-reported questionnaire designed to measure various causes of sexual desire in both male and female participants. It evaluates sexual desire from both dyadic and solitary standpoints, providing deeper insight into the etiology of potential desire disorders.

9.2.2.1 Development and Validation

The SDI was developed to evaluate potential factors that may lead to decreased desire for either partnered or solitary sexual activity. It has undergone two revisions prior to its current state, the SDI-2, which demonstrates good statistical strength, with a Cronbach's α of 0.88 for dyadic sexual desire and 0.91 for solitary sexual desire.

9.2.2.2 Structure and Content

The SDI is a 14-item evaluation that comprises eight questions related to dyadic sexual desire and six relating to solitary sexual desire. These two sections are scored independently, with a higher score representing higher levels of sexual desire. The scores are then compiled to give an overall total desire score.

9.2.2.3 Administration and Use

The SDI is typically self-administered. It takes roughly five minutes to complete, allowing for use in both the clinical and research setting.

9.2.2.4 Applications and Implications

The SDI is used mainly as an indicator of current levels of sexual desire. It can be used to track sexual desire tendencies over time, as well as to evaluate the efficacy of different therapies for low sexual desire.

9.2.2.5 Strengths and Limitations

As it focuses on both solitary and dyadic sexual desire, the SDI is valuable for differentiating when a patient's low desire may be due to partner-related issues. Its ease of use is also a strength of the metric. Much like the FSFI, however, the SDI only considers the past 30 days, which may be of varying usefulness in non–sexually active patients and suffers from the typical limitations of self-reported questionnaires.

9.3 Scales for Assessment of Sexual Arousal

9.3.1 Sexual Arousal and Desire Inventory

The Sexual Arousal and Desire Inventory (SADI)[202] is a multifaceted, descriptor-based inventory that assesses subjective sexual arousal and desire in female and male participants. It was originally designed to evaluate changes in desire and arousal when participants were exposed to erotica.

9.3.1.1 Development and Validation

The SADI was developed to evaluate both arousal and desire, which while often occurring simultaneously, are rarely studied together. It has different iterations that also include potential changes in desire and arousal when exposed to erotic music or music videos. The latest iteration of the SADI demonstrates a Cronbach's α for the Motivational subscale of 0.719 and Cronbach's α for the Physiological subscale of 0.850.

9.3.1.2 Structure and Content

The SADI typically comprises multiple items that assess different dimensions of sexual arousal and desire, including subjective arousal, physiological arousal, sexual interest, and sexual satisfaction. Respondents rate each item based on their own experiences and perceptions, providing a comprehensive evaluation of their sexual arousal and desire.

9.3.1.3 Administration and Use

The SADI utilizes a five-point Likert scale to rate 54 descriptors that apply to the participant's regular sexual desire and arousal, which are then delineated into evaluative, psychological, motivational, and aversion factors. Its use is primarily geared towards research, although it could be incorporated into clinical practice in the preclinical setting.

9.3.1.4 Applications and Implications

As a research tool, the SADI allows researchers to evaluate subjective descriptors that the research subject finds arousing. The subjective nature of the inventory allows for cultural variations, as well as what descriptors lean more towards desire versus arousal.

9.3.1.5 Strengths and Limitations

The main strength of the SADI and its iterations is its evaluation of arousal and desire simultaneously. As it is a research tool, it has applications in the laboratory setting, but is not as useful as a clinical metric. Additionally, since it is subjective in nature, results are susceptible to the traditional biases that accompany subjective questionnaires.

9.4 Scales for Assessment of Orgasm

9.4.1 Orgasm Rating Scale

The Orgasm Rating Scale (ORS)[203] is a metric used to evaluate the subjective experience of orgasm in both male and female individuals. It is based on the Multidimensional Model of the Subjective Experience of Orgasm[204] originally described by Mah and Binik and provides the evaluator with information about the subject's personal experience with both solitary and partnered orgasms.

9.4.1.1 Development and Validation

The ORS was developed to address the lack of comprehensive, theory-based metrics for subjective orgasm experience. It has been validated in multiple languages, and while originally geared towards heterosexual participants, it has been expanded to include specific wording for homosexual individuals. It boasts an internal consistency between 0.78 for the Intimacy domain and 0.93 for the sensory domain. It has also been shown to distinguish between individuals with and without orgasmic dysfunction.

9.4.1.2 Structure and Content

The ORS consists of 40 self-reported questions on an adjective-based scale. It assesses both sensory (physical sensation) and cognitive (satisfaction, intimacy) facets of orgasm, asking the participant to rate adjectives describing their last orgasm on a 0 to 5 scale.

9.4.1.3 Administration and Use

The ORS is designed to be a self-administered questionnaire. It is used primarily in the research setting but could also be used in a clinical role if time permits. It requires approximately five to ten minutes to complete.

9.4.1.4 Applications and Implications

As a research tool, the data gleaned from the ORS can be used to not only provide information about orgasmic experiences but also allow researchers to follow treatment outcomes and medication therapy in terms of their effects on orgasm.

9.4.1.5 Strengths and Limitations

The ORS offers several strengths, including its simplicity, ease of administration, and ability to capture subjective experiences of orgasm. However, its reliance on self-reporting may introduce biases, and its effectiveness may vary depending on the individual's ability to accurately assess and report what sensations and emotions they experience with orgasm.

9.4.2 Female Orgasm Scale

The Female Orgasm Scale (FOS)[205] is a tool used to evaluate both consistency and satisfaction with orgasm during partnered sexual activity. It does not address any facet of orgasm with self-stimulation.

9.4.2.1 Development and Validation

The FOS was developed to provide a quick, easily completable tool that allows for evaluation of orgasmic activity. It has a high internal consistency, with a Cronbach's α of 0.84 to 0.86.

9.4.2.2 Structure and Content

The FOS consists of seven questions. Five questions evaluate orgasmic frequency during various sexual activities (intercourse, oral stimulation, self-stimulation in the presence of a partner, etc.), and two assess satisfaction with orgasm.

9.4.2.3 Administration and Use

The FOS can be self-reported or administered by research/healthcare staff. It takes roughly five minutes to complete and is suitable for use in both research and clinical settings.

9.4.2.4 Applications and Implications

As a research tool, the FOS can provide information on partnered orgasmic issues and has application for monitoring orgasmic changes related to medications or other health-related conditions.

9.4.2.5 Strengths and Limitations

The main strength of the FOS is its brevity and ease of use. Its obvious limitation is its concentration on partnered orgasmic activity only, in addition to the typical limitations encountered with self-reporting metrices.

9.5 Scales for Assessment of Sexual Satisfaction

9.5.1 Index of Sexual Satisfaction

The Index of Sexual Satisfaction (ISS)[206] is a scale used to measure the degree of satisfaction and dissatisfaction in individuals in a current dyadic, sexual relationship.

9.5.1.1 Development and Validation

The ISS was developed to address the need for a reliable and valid measure of sexual satisfaction. It has a Cronbach's α of 0.92 and a standard error of the mean (SEM) of 4.24.

9.5.1.2 Structure and Content

The ISS is composed of 25 questions, each which are rated on a 1 to 7 scale, with test questions 1, 2, 3, 9, 10, 12, 16, 17, 19, 21, 22, and 23 reverse-scored. The ratings are then complied, with a final score between 0 and 100, with higher scores equating higher degrees of dissatisfaction. A score of 30 or less is considered optimal.

9.5.1.3 Administration and Use

The ISS is administered by a researcher or clinician. Due to its ease of use, it can be performed in both the research and clinical setting.

9.5.1.4 Applications and Implications

The ISS is intended to be utilized multiple times over a treatment period to assess for changes associated with sexual satisfaction.

9.5.1.5 Strengths and Limitations

The main strength of the ISS is its brevity and ease of use. Its straight-forward grading system also allows for quick comparison between administrations. Its main limitations are its focus on dyadic sexual satisfaction alone, as well as the fact that it is not readily available without purchase.

9.6 Scales for Assessment of Vaginismus

9.6.1 Multidimensional Vaginal Penetration Disorder Questionnaire

The Multidimensional Vaginal Penetration Disorder Questionnaire (MVPDQ)[207] is a specialized metric designed to assess various dimensions of vaginal penetration difficulties in female participants. It is unique in that it provides a genital diagram for participants to show the location of their pain in addition to a focused questionnaire.

9.6.1.1 Development and Validation

The MVPDQ was developed to assess various psychological factors in unconsummated married individuals with lifelong vaginismus. The metric efficacy was evaluated with exploratory factor analysis, demonstrating a Cronbach's α of 0.79 and test-retest values ranging from 0.78 to 0.87.

9.6.1.2 Structure and Content

The MVPDQ is a self-administered, 72-item questionnaire that evaluates the following topics: catastrophic fears regarding vaginal penetration, pelvic muscle dysfunction/pain during penetration, psychological and relational problems experienced when vaginal penetration fails, sexual information about penetration, knowledge of female and male genital anatomy, hypervigilance/avoidance, marital adjustment, optimism regarding future and treatment, reasons for penetration, and negative thoughts about genital compatibility. When using the anatomic pain chart, the intensity of pain is assessed on a 0 to 3 scale, with each value demonstrating more discomfort.

9.6.1.3 Administration and Use

The MVPDQ is self-administered, with results interpreted by research or clinical personnel. While the questionnaire was developed for married individuals, it can be used in nonmarried participants with vaginismus who desire vaginal penetration.

9.6.1.4 Applications and Implications

The main application for the MVPDQ is in aiding the clinician in the treatment of vaginismus. As previously discussed, vaginismus is often best treated in a multidisciplinary fashion, and the MVPDQ can aid providers in coordinating care teams for patients with penetration disorders.

9.6.1.5 Strengths and Limitations

The main strength of the MVPDQ is its comprehensive nature, as well as its unique anatomic pain map. In the hands of a sexual medicine specialist, these factors can significantly aid in determining the base etiology for the patient's difficulty with penetration. Its main limitations are its length, as well as its reliance on well-trained, knowledgeable providers to assign treatment protocols based on the results of the questionnaire.

9.7 Conclusion

Sexual medicine is a field that is dominated by the subjective. Many of the symptoms or complaints patients describe are purposely not reproduced in the exam room and therefore lack clinically objective measurements often seen in other fields of medicine – one cannot assess the severity of a patient's low sex drive as they would auscultate their lung sounds. Sexual medicine metrics, therefore, are helpful (if not necessary) to monitor and evaluate changes in sexual dysfunction over time. Just as a blood pressure log can determine the efficacy of an antihypertensive drug, so too can repeat applications of a specific sexual medicine metric report improvement in sexual function. While this is obviously useful in the research setting, it is equally helpful for patients to see these changes and may lead to better compliance with medication or therapies.

As stated in the introduction, most electronic medical record programs do not have any of the "regular" sexual medicine metrices incorporated into their software, let alone the more obscure ones. As such, it is important for sexual medicine providers to be knowledgeable about where these metrices may be found. Some are open access and readily available with a quick internet search, while others may be behind paywalls or other proprietary sources. Additionally, many of the metrics previously discussed have gone through multiple iterations or have been adapted into other languages or for other specific demographic groups. The author therefore recommends developing a good relationship with a medical librarian if possible. Finally, much of the information contained in this chapter was found in the citations provided by the open-access article "Assessment Scales for Sexual Disorders – A Review" by Grover and Shoun.[208] Interested readers should review that article for even more in-depth discussions about various sexual medicine metrics and questionnaires.

9.8 Case Study

Elisa is a 28-year-old female who presents to your office complaining of low sex drive. She states that while she enjoys sex, she lacks any desire to initiate it. She denies any other factors that may be contributing to her low desire at this time and reports that her current relationship is very strong. You state that you think a questionnaire may be helpful in determining the cause of her low drive. She responds with, "I don't really have time to fill anything out, but if it's short, I guess I'll do it." Which of the following metrics may be useful in determining the etiology of her sexual concerns?

A: The Sexual Function Questionnaire (SDQ)
B: The Decreased Sexual Desire Screener (DSDS)
C: The Sexual Arousal and Desire Inventory (SADI)
D: All of the above

The answer is B. The DSDS is a short five-question screening tool specifically designed to assess for HSDD. The SDQ is a multifactorial questionnaire that, while it includes questions about desire, focuses more on multiple domains of sexual function. The SADI does address desire, but is intended more for research and is not as applicable in a clinical setting.

Chapter 10

The Effects of Lifestyle Factors on Female Sexual Function

If we look at sexuality from a basic science standpoint, it is easy to distill it into purely an interplay between hormones, neurotransmitters, and various physiologic changes – a type of Newtonian Rube Goldberg creation where one action leads to a very specific reaction. While this may be true on an incredibly basic level, the reality is that sexual function – and sexuality in general – requires weaving multiple lifestyle factors together to create a vibrant tapestry of sexual health. And much like a real-life tapestry, enough tension on any one strand may lead to an unraveling of the entire creation.

In an effort to more fully understand the nonmedical aspects of sexuality, researchers have begun to evaluate various lifestyle factors as they relate to sexual function. While it may seem obvious that, for instance, chronic fatigue may lead to a lack of sexual desire, it is not as clear-cut as to whether a sedentary lifestyle may cause dyspareunia or whether work-related stressors may lead to orgasmic dysfunction. As such, it is important for the sexual medicine provider to fully understand the ways in which lifestyle factors can affect sexuality and be able to provide recommendations outside of pharmaceuticals and therapy when needed.

In this chapter, we will focus on the roles of various lifestyle choices such as nutrition, exercise, and stress management and discuss the possible implications those factors have on sexual function. We will also discuss specific psychosocial factors, such as emotional wellbeing, past trauma, and body image. It

DOI: 10.1201/9781003494522-10

must be understood that this chapter is not designed to be an end-all-be-all treatise on sexual function and lifestyle factors but should instead be viewed as an introduction to those connections, as well as a reminder to look holistically at patients when discussing sexual concerns. Table 10.1 sets out the lifestyle factors to be discussed further.

10.1 The Role of Nutrition, Exercise, and Activity on Female Sexual Function

It is common knowledge that food and activity affect how we feel. This concept is not a new one – Hippocrates wrote, "Let food be thy medicine and medicine be thy food," in the 4th century BCE, and dietary cuneiform tablets from ancient Babylon show well-balanced recipes of stews made with a variety of meats, vegetables, and spices.[209] Even the idiom "you are what you eat" harkens to the idea that health is invariably connected to our diet. Similarly, no respected professional health organization would refute the statement "activity and exercise are beneficial for health." As a species, we simply feel better when we are able to move, and as bodybuilder Eugen Sandow once said, "Life is movement. Once you stop moving, you're dead."

The connection between diet, activity, and sexual function is no less robust – and this makes sense. If a patient presents to the clinic appearing malnourished and ill, it is logical to assume that their sexual functioning is not going to be optimum. From an evolutionary perspective, sex, especially if it leads to conception, requires a significant investment in terms of energy and resources for the female participant. In a low energy/nutrient state, therefore, the body will preserve homeostatic functions first and only allow the expenditure of (sexual) resources if all other needs are filled. Likewise, an individual bedbound due to illness or injury may not have a desire to engage in sexual activity until they feel better and are able to better move throughout space. Additionally, chronic illness as a whole may lead to muscle wasting or, conversely, contracture or spasm and may make engaging in sexual activity almost impossible due to pain or lack of stamina. As such, it behooves the sexual medicine provider to address these lifestyle factors when evaluating a patient.

10.1.1 Dietary Factors and Female Sexual Function

The standard American diet (SAD), with its high intake of highly processed foods, refined carbohydrates, added sugars, industrially processed meats, and high-fat dairy products, is directly linked to numerous health issues, such as hypertension and diabetes, not to mention sexual concerns such as low sex drive and arousal disorders in both men and women.[210,211] On the

TABLE 10.1 Quick Reference: Lifestyle Factors and Sexual Function

Lifestyle Factor	Effects on Desire	Effects on Arousal	Effects on Pain	Effects on Orgasm
Nutrition/Amino acids	Varied diet shows positive effect on desire. Nutrient deficiencies – zinc, arginine, L–citrulline – associated with low drive.	Excessive or restricted caloric intake linked to arousal dysfunction.	Excessive intake of inflammatory foods may increase pain. Possible connection between gut dysbiosis and pain.	Foods that increase NO may help with orgasmic dysfunction.
Nutraceuticals/Supplements	Tentative correlation, data is relatively lacking.	NO boosters may help with arousal dysfunction.	Phytoestrogens, collagen synthesis may help reduce pain from GSM, vaginal dryness.	Phytoestrogens and NO boosters may improve orgasmic dysfunction.
General activity and exercise	Exercise-related improvement in body image may improve sexual desire.	Strong correlation between exercise and a reduction in arousal dysfunctions.	Increase in activity and mobility found to be protective against sexual pain.	Improved pelvic floor function strength associated with decrease in orgasmic dysfunction.
Sleep changes	Sleep deficit connected to decreased levels of desire and arousal.	Sleep deficit connected to decreased levels of desire	Chronic sleep deprivation correlates with decreased tolerance to pain.	No specific correlation noted.
Stress management	High stress connected to HSDD, SAD.	Reduction in stress improved FSAD.	Stress reduction techniques improve pain in patients with PFD.	Stress reduction associated with improvement in anorgasmia.
Psychosocial factors: Emotional wellbeing	Significant association between depression, anxiety, and desire disorders.	Increased anxiety associated with decrease in sexual arousal.	Depression linked to greater manifestation of vulvodynia. Improved emotional wellbeing protective against PFD.	Dysorgasmia and anorgasmia both correlated with poor emotional state. PDOD directly linked to emotional wellbeing.
Psychosocial factors: Previous sexual trauma	Strongly associated with female sexual dysfunction of all types.			
Psychosocial factors: Body image	Poor body image associated with decrease in overall desire.	Anxiety about body image correlated to FSAD.	Better body image protective against dyspareunia.	Lower body image associated with increased risk for FOD.

contrary, a varied diet, especially one similar to those found in geographic "blue zones," is associated with overall longevity and decreased morbidity,[212] and data has shown that a healthy diet also correlates with improved sexual function,[213] with patients reporting higher levels of libido and sexual satisfaction when consuming a diet rich in nuts, fruits, leafy greens, and fish with high omega-3 concentrations.[214] In fact, multiple studies have determined that following the Mediterranean diet results in increased sexual function in a dose-dependent manner regardless of menopausal status or presence of metabolic disease. It appears that the healthiest style of eating for sexual wellbeing – along with general health and wellness – is one that prioritizes plants and whole foods.

Outside of specific diets, it is also important to note that caloric restriction, whether through dieting or fasting, especially in combination with a low body weight, can have a negative effect on sexual function. This is likely due to a combination of endocrine dysregulation and psychological factors stemming from a decrease in cholesterol-based steroid sex hormones and possible body dysmorphias. As such, the sexual medicine provider must be aware of these factors when discussing sexual health with patients. Questions such as "Tell me about your diet" or "What type of foods do you enjoy eating?" are open-ended and nonthreatening and can allow the clinician to gain insight into the dietary patterns of the patient. Moreover, physical exam findings that are associated with eating disorders, such as the presence of lanugo hair, dental carries, callouses on the dorsum of the hand associated with self-induced vomiting, or overall signs of cachexia, may point towards a much more concerning underlying condition such as anorexia or bulimia nervosa, with the presenting sexual concern simply being a symptom of the disease.

In addition to dietary choices, it is important for the clinician to ask about supplement, vitamin, and herbal therapy usage when discussing sexual concerns. In February 2021, the National Center for Health Statistics reported that during 2018 over 57.6% of Americans used some form of supplement and that older Americans were more likely to use more supplements than their younger counterparts.[215] Furthermore, a report from the American Urologic Association in 2022 stated the global sexual health supplement market is expected to reach $608 million by 2030.[216] It is imperative, therefore, that the sexual medicine provider be familiar with most of the more routine vitamins, supplements, and herbs that are associated with sexual function.

Table 10.2 lists known (and theoretical) correlations between supplement therapy and the individual domains of sexual function. It should be stated that the field of wellness-based sexual medicine is burgeoning at best and the amount of research on specific supplements in terms of sexual function is sparse, especially for female patients. Additionally, no set dosing regimen

TABLE 10.2 Nutrient Effects on Sexual Function

Nutrient	Source	Suspected Mechanism of Action	Sexual Function Domains Possibly Addressed	Usual Dosage/ Frequency
Amino Acids				
L-Arginine	Red meat, poultry, fish, dairy, nuts, seeds, legumes	Precursor to nitric oxide, helps improve blood flow and vascular function	Desire, arousal orgasm[217]	2–6 grams per day
L-Citrulline	Watermelon, cucumbers, some melons	Converted into L-arginine in the kidneys, thereby increasing blood flow	Arousal, orgasm	3–6 grams per day
D-Aspartic acid	Meat, eggs, dairy (though supplementation is more common)	Increases luteinizing hormone (LH) levels, which may boost testosterone production	Desire, arousal, orgasm	2–3 grams per day
L-Taurine	Meat, fish, dairy, energy drinks	Interacts with GABA receptors, possibly producing calming effect	Desire, arousal	500 mg to 3 grams per day
L-Glutamine/glutamate	Meat, fish, eggs, dairy, spinach, cabbage	Affects NMDA receptors,[218] which regulate release of dopamine and other neurotransmitters	Desire	5–15 grams per day
Herbal Supplements				
Maca (*Lepidium meyenii*)	Root native to Peru	Suspected sexual effect from phytosterols or phytoestrogens	Desire[219]	1.5–6 grams per day
Damiana (*Turnera diffusa*)	Leaf from a shrub native to Central and South America	Flavonoids may exert alpha 2-adrenergic receptor antagonism, increasing blood flow[220]	Arousal, orgasm[221]	400–800 mg of extract per day

(Continued)

TABLE 10.2 (Continued) Nutrient Effects on Sexual Function

Nutrient	Source	Suspected Mechanism of Action	Sexual Function Domains Possibly Addressed	Usual Dosage/Frequency
Tribulus terrestris	Plant found in Mediterranean regions, Africa, Asia	May enhance testosterone levels by increasing DHEA synthesis[222]	Desire, arousal, orgasm[223]	250–750 mg per day
Panax ginseng spp.	Root native to Korea, northeastern China, and Siberia	Thought to enhance nitric oxide synthesis	Arousal, orgasm[224]	200–1000 mg of extract per day
Yohimbine (often confused with yohimbe) (*Pausinystalia johimbe*)	Bark from an evergreen tree native to Central Africa	Alpha-2 adrenergic receptors antagonist increases genital blood flow	Arousal, orgasm	5–15 mg of yohimbine per day
Horny goat weed (*Epimedium grandiflorum*)	Leaf from a plant found in China and Asia	Contains icariin, which inhibits PDE5, leading to vasodilation	Arousal, orgasm	500–1000 mg of extract per day
Fenugreek (*Trigonella* spp.)	Seeds from a plant native to the Mediterranean, southern Europe, and western Asia	Saponins in seeds thought to increase estradiol and testosterone production[225]	Desire, arousal, pain, orgasm	500–600 mg of extract per day
Ashwagandha (*Withania somnifera*)	Root from a plant native to India, Middle East, Africa	Thought to increase testosterone production and decrease cortisol levels[226]	Desire,[227] arousal, orgasm	300–500 mg of extract standardized to withanolides
Gingko biloba	Leaves from the ginkgo tree native to China	Increases blood flow and nitric oxide activity	Desire, arousal[228]	120–300 mg of extract per day
Soy (*Glycine max*)	Beans from the soy plant, found in East Asia	Known phytoestrogenic activity – may increase vaginal blood flow, lubrication, and vaginal collagen content	Desire, arousal, pain	15–25 grams per day of soy protein and/or 50–100 mg per day of isoflavones

Slippery elm (*Ulmus rubra*)	Bark from the slippery elm tree native to North America	May increase lubrication in mucosal tissues throughout the body	Arousal, pain	400–1000 mg of bark powder per day
Vitamins and Minerals				
Vitamin A	Carrots, sweet potatoes, spinach, and dairy products	Affects mucous membranes, important for sex steroid formation	Desire, arousal, orgasm	Recommended daily allowance (RDA): • 700 mcg per day
Vitamin B complex (3, 6, 12)	Meat, fish, poultry, fortified cereals, and legumes	Affect metabolism and neurotransmitter production, important for cellular oxygen transport	Desire,[229] arousal	RDA: • 14 mg per day (B_3) • 1.5 mg per day (B_6) • 2.4 mcg per day (B_{12})
Vitamin C	Citrus fruits, strawberries, bell peppers, and broccoli	Necessary for collagen synthesis[230]	Arousal, pain	RDA: • 75 mg per day
Vitamin D	Fatty fish, fortified milk, and exposure to sunlight	Vitamin D receptors are present in ovarian and genital tissue and facilitate the production of sex steroids[231] Vitamin D also necessary for dopamine activity	Desire, arousal, pain, orgasm	RDA: • 600 IU (15 mcg) per day for women under 70 • 800 IU (20 mcg) for women aged 70+
Vitamin E	Vegetable oils, nuts, seeds, and leafy greens	Affects lipid membrane packaging, reduces local inflammation	Arousal, pain	RDA: • 15 mg per day
Zinc	Meat, shellfish, legumes, seeds, and nuts	Required for testosterone production and synthesis from LH[232]	Desire, arousal, pain, orgasm[233]	RDA: • 8 mg per day

(Continued)

TABLE 10.2 (*Continued*) Nutrient Effects on Sexual Function

Nutrient	Source	Suspected Mechanism of Action	Sexual Function Domains Possibly Addressed	Usual Dosage/ Frequency
Magnesium	Green leafy vegetables, nuts, seeds, whole grains, and legumes	Necessary for sex steroid synthesis, especially testosterone Estrogenic effects enhanced by magnesium[234]	Desire, arousal	RDA: • 310–320 mg per day
Iodine	Iodized salt, seafood, dairy products, and eggs	Required for appropriate thyroid function	Desire, arousal	RDA: • 150 mcg per day
Sodium	Salt tablets	Excessive sodium intake associated with vasoconstriction	Arousal	RDA: • 1500 mg per day (upper limit: 2300 mg per day)
Iron	Red meat, poultry, lentils, and fortified cereals	Required for heme synthesis and oxygen transport Iron deficiency associated with sexual dysfunction[235]	Desire, arousal, pain, orgasm	RDA: • 18 mg per day for women aged under 50 • 8 mg for women 51+

exists for dietary supplements or herbal therapies. The values listed here are considered "safe" overall but may not be appropriate for any given patient. Furthermore, as regulation for supplements and herbal therapies is limited at best, the quality of the ingredients may also be suspect and may lead to varying results. The author recommends consulting with a registered nutritional specialist for supplement recommendations and a registered herbalist for herbal therapies if they wish to provide supplements as treatment options for their patients. A naturopathic physician (ND) can also be a resource for these types of therapies, as their training includes both supplements and herbal medicine. The following list is by no means exhaustive but provides a basic overview of possible nutraceutical therapies for patients with sexual concerns.

10.1.2 Activity and Exercise and Female Sexual Function

As stated in the Introduction, physical activity and sexual function are inextricably linked, with almost all bodily systems benefiting from regular exercise. Cardiovascular health is especially important for sexual function, as sexual activity leads to a statistically significant increase in overall heart rate and blood pressure,[236] which, as discussed in Chapter 4, is essential for sexual arousal. Recall that the increase in blood flow to the genitalia not only provides engorgement of the labia and clitoris but also increases vaginal transudate, providing natural lubrication for penetrative activity. In patients with impaired cardiovascular health, sexual dysfunction is a common symptom, with arousal disorders being especially prevalent.

For patients transitioning through menopause, the importance of exercise becomes even more pronounced. Hormonal changes during perimenopause and menopause can lead to decreased libido, vaginal dryness, and weight gain, all of which may significantly impact sexual satisfaction.[237] In addition to conventional therapy, regular physical activity can alleviate many of these symptoms by improving mood and overall body composition, with strength training being additionally beneficial for combating age-related muscle loss and improving bone density. Weight loss in general has been found to be helpful in improving function, with one study demonstrating a loss of more than 5% of body weight yielding an overall improvement in Female Sexual Function Index (FSFI) score by 3 points.[238]

So, what type of exercise is best? While the connection between exercise and sexual function is well established, the specific impact of various forms of exercise is still being studied.[239] Aerobic exercises, resistance/weight training, and mind-body activities like yoga or Pilates each offer unique benefits to sexual health, depending on a woman's life stage, fitness level, and overall wellbeing. Further research is needed, however, to explore how different types of exercise can be tailored to improve specific aspects of sexual function, particularly in certain populations such as postmenopausal patients or those dealing with chronic health conditions. As the understanding of these relationships evolves and research continues to be performed, healthcare providers will be better equipped to offer personalized recommendations that support both general and sexual health.

10.2 The Effect of Sleep and Stress on Female Sexual Function

Sleep and stress are two critical factors that significantly impact female sexual function. It is a well-established fact that poor sleep quality is linked to various health issues such as hypertension and dyslipidemia,[240] but its connection to sexual health is often overlooked. Women who experience sleep disturbances such as insomnia or poor-quality sleep report higher levels of sexual dysfunction, including issues with desire, arousal, and overall satisfaction.[241] This may be due to the connection between the suprachiasmatic nucleus in the hypothalamus, which regulates sleep patterns, and its connection to the hypothalamic–pituitary–adrenal (HPA) axis, which governs stress response.[242] If sleep is consistently disrupted, the resulting overproduction of stress hormones may create an inhibitory effect on gonadal estradiol and testosterone. Furthermore, sex hormone secretion is intrinsically tied to our circadian rhythms, and as such, persistently abnormal sleep patterns can lead to an overall reduction in sex hormone release.[243]

Finally, chronic sleep deprivation is associated with decreased pain tolerance. It is estimated that 67% to 88% of individuals with chronic pain experience sleep disruption and insomnia and at least 50% of people with insomnia report chronic pain.[244] Given that roughly 70% of individuals with chronic pain also report some form of sexual dysfunction,[245] it is imperative that proper sleep hygiene be discussed when patients report both chronic pain and sexual concerns. Accordingly, Table 10.3 gives the recommendations from the Sleep Foundation[246] to achieve optimum sleeping habits.

In a similar fashion, stress, whether acute or chronic, has an equally profound effect on female sexual function. As previously stated, stress activates the HPA axis, leading to the release of cortisol, the body's primary stress hormone. Moreover, chronic stress has a direct impact on the brain's ability to regulate emotional and physical responses during sexual activity, as high levels of stress over time can impair the brain's reward systems via the effect of cortisol on the limbic system.[247] In the presence of elevated cortisol, dopamine production is diminished, which leads to a decline in motivation for pleasure-seeking activities such as sex. Additionally, low dopamine can also disrupt communication between the brain and body, leading to a lower sensitivity to sexual stimuli and reduced satisfaction. Finally, chronic stress is associated with cognitive distractions as well, which in turn may lead to

TABLE 10.3 Sleep Hygiene Suggestions

Invest in a better mattress and bedding	Block out lights	Get at least 7–8 hours of sleep
Minimize noise	Set alarm for same time every day	Relax 30 minutes before bed
Set thermostat to 65–68 degrees	Keep naps to 20 minutes	Disconnect devices the hour before bed
Limit caffeine after 2 p.m.	Get 30 minutes of natural light exposure	Exercise for at least 20 minutes a day
Be mindful of alcohol in the hour before bedtime	Eat dinner a few hours before bed	Limit nicotine use and smoke exposure
Reserve bed for sleep and sex only	Get out of bed after 20 minutes if you have difficulty falling asleep	Keep a sleep diary
Consider supplements to help with sleep	Talk with a sleep specialist	

problems with psychological arousal or a sense of "not being there" during sexual activity. As such, it is no wonder that patients experiencing chronic stress are more likely to report a bevy of sexual concerns, including problems with desire, arousal, and orgasm.[248]

Unfortunately, this interplay between sleep and stress creates a vicious cycle. Poor sleep exacerbates stress levels, while chronic stress leads to sleep disturbances, both of which negatively affect sexual function. This bidirectional relationship suggests that treatment approaches need to address both stress management and sleep improvement to effectively treat female sexual dysfunction. Recognizing the dual impact of these lifestyle factors allows the sexual medicine provider to adopt more comprehensive strategies to improve the outcomes for their patients.

10.3 The Roles of Emotional Wellbeing, Sexual Trauma, and Body Image on Female Sexual Function

Emotional wellbeing is intrinsically tied to sexuality, as individuals experiencing anxiety, depression, or even low self-esteem often experience sexual concerns.[249] The inverse of this fact is also true, as patients with stronger psychological health often report better sexual function overall. Research even supports the idea of "sexual resiliency," a concept indicating that individuals with higher emotional resilience tend to experience fewer sexual difficulties.[250,251] For this reason, discussing emotional coping strategies can be a crucial part of the conversation between sexual medicine providers and their patients.

TABLE 10.4 Coping Styles and Strategies

Coping Style	Guiding Questions	Example Questions
Problem-focused	Do you think this is something you can control? What actions can you take to help resolve the problem?	What treatments could you explore that would help reduce your pain with intercourse?
Emotion-focused	How are you feeling about this situation? What makes you feel more relaxed when you are upset?	What can you do to help manage your anxiety before sexual activity?
Meaning-focused	How has this experience strengthened you, even though it is difficult? What can you learn from this?	How can this challenge be a new way of exploring intimacy?
Avoidance	What would happen if you faced this problem directly, instead of avoiding it? What distractions are you using to keep from addressing the problem?	What do you fear might happen if you talk to your partner about your sexual concerns?

Four main coping styles are traditionally recognized: problem-focused, emotion-focused, meaning-focused, and avoidance. In practice, these coping styles can manifest in unique ways for patients with sexual dysfunction. Some may prefer problem-solving approaches, seeking direct solutions to their challenges, while others might find relief in exploring the emotional roots of their concerns. Patients often employ a mix of these strategies when dealing with stressors, and by identifying which strategies resonate with each patient, providers can offer tailored advice or refer them to mental health specialists such as sex therapists.

That said, for many non–mental health providers, discussing emotional coping strategies may feel outside their professional comfort zone. However, opening the conversation with simple, guiding questions can create a bridge for further dialogue. These initial discussions can help patients reflect on how they cope with their sexual concerns and may pave the way for more in-depth exploration with a therapist or counselor. Table 10.4 lists potential guiding questions, as well as examples, to help patients think about possible coping strategies.

10.3.1 Previous Sexual Trauma and Its Impact on Sexual Health

Previous sexual trauma can have a profound impact on a person's sexual health. Even if a patient is not officially diagnosed with posttraumatic stress disorder (PTSD), the effects of the traumatic experience can be long-lasting and can affect sexual function on both a conscious and subconscious level. From a neuroscientific perspective, trauma induces changes in three critical areas of the brain – the prefrontal cortex, the amygdala, and the hippocampus. These regions control rational thought, emotional processing, and memory differentiation between past and present, respectively. When a trauma survivor experiences a situation or event similar to a previously traumatic one, the brain can have a difficult time differentiating it from the previous trauma. As such, survivors of sexual trauma act negatively in a safe sexual situation, experiencing fear, anxiety, or distress.

The statistics around trauma and sexual dysfunction are sobering, with roughly 80% of female patients with a history of childhood sexual trauma reporting sexual concerns as an adult.[252] Additionally, 71% to 88% of victims of rape and sexual assault encounter issues with sexual function.[253] Patients often report challenges with desire and satisfaction, though any domain of sexual function can be affected. Furthermore, survivors may experience feelings of shame, hypervigilance during sexual activity, and emotional numbness,[254] while others may experience chronic pelvic pain, pelvic floor dysfunction, or dyspareunia.[255,256]

Despite these challenges, recovery from sexual trauma is possible. Utilizing a multidisciplinary care approach, including trauma therapy and sex therapy, the sexual medicine provider can help patients with a history of sexual trauma achieve their sexual goals. Furthermore, trauma-focused therapies such as cognitive behavioral therapy (CBT) or eye movement desensitization and reprocessing (EMDR) can lead to significant improvements in overall sexual function, especially if combined with appropriate medical interventions. Finally, supportive, open communication with partners, as well as the creation of a safe space for healing, can help rebuild sexual confidence. As always, the sexual medicine provider must remember that each approach should be individualized and counsel patients properly that healing from sexual trauma is not a "quick fix," but rather something that may take a significant amount of time and emotional investment

10.3.2 Body Image and Female Sexual Function

The interplay between sex and body image predates civilization itself. Even in the animal kingdom, species that reproduce sexually often select mates based on physical traits and characteristics that will better benefit the species. In humans, however, sexual attraction extends beyond procreation; our perceived attractiveness and how we think others view us significantly influence our own sexual behavior. According to an *Allure* magazine reader survey, more than 64% of people report that physical attraction is important when choosing a mate, and over half of people surveyed reported that they were defined by their physical appearance.[257] It comes as no surprise, therefore, that how we perceive our *physical self* plays a pivotal role in shaping our *sexual self.*

The ideal body has long been a source of discussion, and what is beautiful in one part of the world may be less so in another. It comes as no surprise, therefore, that cultural factors can idealize certain body types, which often provokes feelings of inadequacy in those who appear different. Research has found that body image dissatisfaction can begin at an early age, with one study demonstrating body image concerns in preschool-aged children, with comments from teachers or parents about physical appearance leading to emotional distress.[258] As we age, these feelings of inadequacy may develop into a highly critical sense of self, including a poor body image. Furthermore, a poor body image may affect multiple aspects of a person's life, including how they perform at work, how they interact without others, and even how they view their own self-worth.[259] These concerns about body image may be heightened during sexual activity, with patients who feel dissatisfied with their bodies experiencing anxiety during sex, focusing on perceived physical flaws, or avoiding sexual activity all together. With continued negative reinforcement, this self-perception can create psychological barriers that affect desire, arousal, and orgasm. In fact, patients with negative body image tend to experience heightened overall sexual distress, which can perpetuate a cycle of body image–induced sexual dissatisfaction.[260]

That said, while research has found that negative body image is associated with decreased desire as well as orgasmic dysfunction, a positive body image correlates with overall enhanced sexual satisfaction.[261] This connection was even further reinforced by Horvath, who demonstrated a direct link between body image satisfaction and greater satisfaction with partnered sexual activity.[262] As such, improving body image through body-positive practices, such as mindfulness, exercise, or therapy, can significantly enhance sexual confidence and satisfaction. Patients who embrace a more positive self-perception are more likely to engage in sexual activity with reduced anxiety, and partners who reinforce body positivity and offer reassurance can also contribute to improving their partner's body image. It is important, therefore, for the sexual medicine provider to address body image concerns as part of a holistic approach to sexual health. When patients with body image concerns have been identified, working in tandem with both mental health professionals, nutritionists, and even life coaches may be able to improve patient outcomes overall. By fostering a positive relationship with their bodies, patients can minimize self-limiting beliefs and embrace a more fulfilling, authentic sexual expression that nurtures both personal and relational well-being.

10.4 Conclusion

The connection between lifestyle choices and sexual health is undeniable. Factors such as physical activity, stress management, and balanced nutrition can not only improve general wellbeing but also contribute to a healthier, more satisfying sexual life. This perspective is essential for the sexual medicine provider. Overall wellness contributes to a positive sexual experience. The opposite is also true. The patient presenting with low desire may suffer from poor nutrition and lack of sleep, while the patient with dyspareunia may have a history of traumatic sexual assault. It is all too easy for the practicing clinician to forget the emotional and spiritual component of the traditional mind-body-spirit triad of overall wellness and instead solely focus on what is occurring on the purely physical level. As such, the author would like to put forth a hierarchy of sexual needs (Figure 10.1) based off the well-known model by Maslow.[263]

In the hierarchy of sexual needs, **physical wellbeing** forms the foundation, as it is the prerequisite for all other levels of sexual function. Proper nutrition, regular exercise, and overall physical care are crucial for maintaining energy, hormonal regulation, and general health, which directly influence a person's sexual health. Moving upward, **emotional wellbeing** must be achieved, as stress, anxiety, and poor mental health can inhibit arousal, desire, and overall sexual satisfaction. Next, addressing **sexual pain** is necessary, as when a patient experiences freedom from sexual pain, they are better equipped to engage in and enjoy sexual activity without fear of discomfort. This in turn allows for **adequate psychological and physiological arousal**, which primes the body and mind for sex, making it possible to experience **heightened sexual desire and interest**

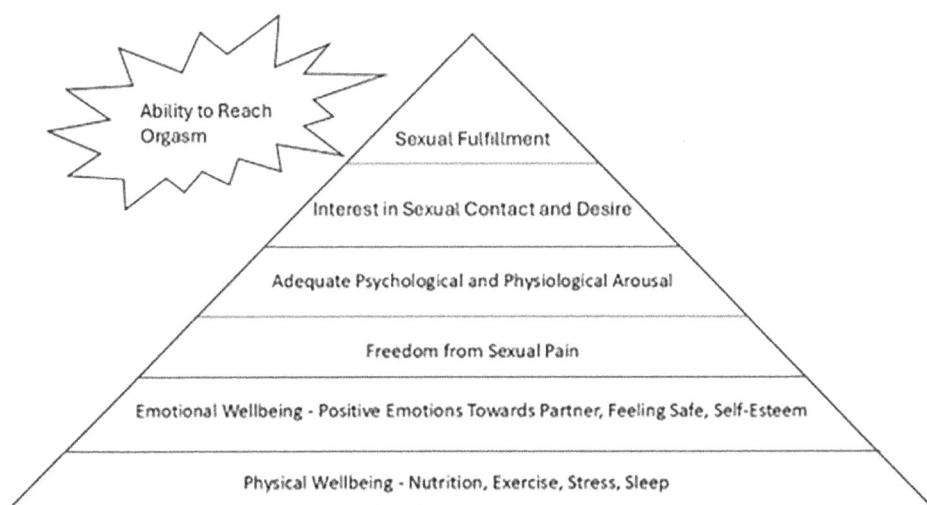

FIGURE 10.1   Hierarchy of sexual needs.

in sexual contact. The culmination of these interconnected needs is **sexual fulfillment**, the highest level of the pyramid, where individuals feel emotionally and physically satisfied in their sexual experiences. The **ability to reach orgasm** exists outside the pyramid, as sexual fulfillment is entirely possible without orgasm. That said, the ability to orgasm also depends on meeting the preceding goals and can be intrinsically tied to overall sexual fulfillment.

As such, by addressing the hierarchy of sexual needs, the sexual medicine provider can help guide patients toward achieving their overall sexual goals, gaining a more fulfilling and satisfying sexual experience, free from concerns or dysfunction, that honors both physical and emotional health. This comprehensive and holistic approach ensures that each level of the hierarchy is acknowledged and paves the way for patients to cultivate a positive relationship with their sexual self.

10.5 Case Study

Emily is a 42-year-old G5P4104 who presents to the clinic wanting to discuss her sexual health. She has recently been diagnosed with a chronic illness and wonders how it may affect her overall sexual function. She states that she often feels tired and that she has difficulty sleeping. She does report that sex is enjoyable for her and denies any concerns with arousal or sexual pain, but worries that her new prescribed medications may affect her libido. She states that she has heard about different herbal therapies for low sex drive and would like to know if there are any specific regimens you could recommend. In addition, she states that she would like to exercise more but feels that her fatigue may limit the amount of exercise that she can do. Which of the following treatment options would you recommend?

A: Improved sleep hygiene, including appropriate bedroom temperature and curtains
B: Consultation with a registered herbalist and strength and conditioning coach
C: Ask about different coping strategies for her newly diagnosed illness
D: All of the above

The answer is D. Discussing sleep hygiene can be a simple and noninvasive recommendation for any patient with sleep problems. Unless the provider has additional training in areas such as herbal medicine, nutrition, or exercise science, referring to a specialist in those areas can be extremely beneficial in assisting the patient to achieve their goals. Finally, the diagnosis of a chronic illness can be difficult for patients to hear. Asking about coping strategies can start a discussion that, if desired, can then pave the way for them to start a relationship with a mental health provider.

Appendix 1

Sexual Medicine Centers

The following is a list of sexual medicine centers in the United States organized alphabetically. While there are undoubtedly other centers not listed here, these have earned recognition for their commitment to providing high-quality sexual medicine care for individuals assigned female at birth. The author also acknowledges that there are many reputable centers outside of the United States but cannot provide commentary on specific international locations. For those seeking providers worldwide, the author recommends visiting the public directory available on the International Society for the Study of Women's Sexual Health website at www.isswsh.org.

Cleveland Clinic Women's Health Clinic
Location: Cleveland, OH
Website: https://my.clevelandclinic.org

Fosnight Center for Sexual Health
Location: Asheville, NC
Website: https://fosnightcenter.com

George Washington Sexual Health and Gender Affirmation Center
NW Washington, DC
Website: https://gwdocs.com/specialties/sexual-health-and-gender-affirmation-center

Haven Center, LLC
Location: Tulsa, OK
Website: www.havencenter.com

IntiMedicine
Location: Washington, DC
Website: https://intimmedicine.com

Mayo Clinic Women's Health Clinic
Location: Rochester, MN
Website: www.mayoclinic.org

Northwestern Medicine Center for Sexual Medicine and Menopause
Location: Chicago, IL
Website: www.nm.org

Rachel Rubin, MD
Location: Washington, DC
Website: www.rachelrubinmd.com

San Diego Sexual Medicine
Location: San Diego, CA
Website: http://sandiegosexualmedicine.com

The Center for Vulvovaginal Disorders
Location: Washington, DC; New York, NY; Tampa, FL
Website: https://vulvodynia.com

UCSF Center for Sexual Health
Location: San Francisco, CA
Website: www.ucsfhealth.org

University of Michigan Women's Sexual Health Program
Location: Ann Arbor, MI
Website: www.uofmhealth.org

UT Southwestern Medical Center – Center for Female Sexual Medicine
Location: Dallas, TX
Website: https://utswmed.org

Women's Health Collective
Location: Grand Rapids, MI
Website: www.whcollective.com

Appendix 2

Release of Health Information Authorization Form

This authorization allows the following institution/provider to release my individually identifiable health information as outlined below. By signing this document, I hereby give my consent for the indicated records to be released.

Patient Information:
Patient Name: _____
Date of Birth: _____

Receiving Clinic/Provider:
Clinic Name: _____
Provider Name: _____
Fax Number: _____
Phone Number: _____
Address: _____
_____

Records to Be Released:
(Please check the types of records to be released)
☐ Clinical Records
☐ Laboratory Data
☐ Imaging Studies
☐ Other: _____

Releasing Clinic Information:

Clinic Name: _____

Fax Number: _____

Signature:

By signing below, I acknowledge that I have read and understand this form. I authorize the release of my medical records as indicated above.

Patient Signature: _____

Date: _____

Appendix 3

Examination Template

Groin:
- ☐ Excoriations
- ☐ Erythematous plaques
- ☐ Stellate papules/pustules
- ☐ Lesions
- ☐ Thickening
- ☐ Ulcerations
- ☐ Masses/nodules
- ☐ Tenderness
- ☐ Loss of sensation
- ☐ Other: _____

Inguinal Crease:
- ☐ Excoriations
- ☐ Ulcerations
- ☐ Pigment changes
- ☐ Lesions
- ☐ Thickening
- ☐ Atrophy
- ☐ Masses/nodules
- ☐ Tenderness
- ☐ Loss of sensation
- ☐ Other: _____

Mons Pubis:
- ☐ Excoriations
- ☐ Ulcerations
- ☐ Pigment changes
- ☐ Lesions
- ☐ Hair changes
- ☐ Masses/nodules
- ☐ Tenderness
- ☐ Loss of sensation
- ☐ Other: _____

Labia Minora:
- ☐ Excoriations
- ☐ Ulcerations
- ☐ Pigment changes
- ☐ Lesions
- ☐ Vesicles
- ☐ Atrophy
- ☐ Masses/nodules
- ☐ Tenderness
- ☐ Loss of sensation
- ☐ Other: _____

Clitoris:
- ☐ Phimosis
- ☐ Ulcerations
- ☐ Pigment changes
- ☐ Lesions
- ☐ Adhesions
- ☐ Atrophy
- ☐ Keratin pearls
- ☐ Tenderness
- ☐ Loss of sensation
- ☐ Other: _____

Posterior Commissure:
- ☐ Fissure
- ☐ Ulcerations
- ☐ Pigment changes
- ☐ Lesions
- ☐ Masses/nodules
- ☐ Tenderness
- ☐ Loss of sensation
- ☐ Other: _____

Anterior Vestibule:
- ☐ Inflammation
- ☐ Ulcerations
- ☐ Pigment changes
- ☐ Lesions
- ☐ Hyperemia
- ☐ Cystic masses
- ☐ Tenderness
- ☐ Loss of sensation
- ☐ Other: _____

Urethra:
- ☐ Caruncle
- ☐ Ulcerations
- ☐ Pigment changes
- ☐ Lesions
- ☐ Masses/nodules
- ☐ Tenderness
- ☐ Loss of sensation
- ☐ Other: _____

Skene's Glands:
- ☐ Erythema
- ☐ Lesions
- ☐ Masses/nodules
- ☐ Tenderness
- ☐ Loss of sensation
- ☐ Other: _____

Posterior Vestibule:
- ☐ Inflammation
- ☐ Pigment changes
- ☐ Lesions
- ☐ Masses/nodules
- ☐ Tenderness
- ☐ Loss of sensation
- ☐ Other: _____

Posterior Fourchette:
- ☐ Fissure
- ☐ Ulcerations
- ☐ Pigment changes
- ☐ Lesions
- ☐ Masses/nodules
- ☐ Tenderness
- ☐ Loss of sensation
- ☐ Other: _____

Bartholin Glands:
- ☐ Lesions
- ☐ Masses/nodules
- ☐ Tenderness
- ☐ Loss of sensation
- ☐ Other: _____

Anterior Vaginal Wall:
- ☐ Ulcerations
- ☐ Prolapse
- ☐ Lesions
- ☐ Atrophy
- ☐ Masses/nodules
- ☐ Tenderness
- ☐ Other: _____

Posterior Vaginal Wall:
- ☐ Ulceration
- ☐ Prolapse
- ☐ Lesions
- ☐ Atrophy
- ☐ Masses/nodules
- ☐ Tenderness
- ☐ Other: _____

Apex:
- ☐ Ulcerations
- ☐ Prolapse
- ☐ Lesions
- ☐ Atrophy
- ☐ Masses/nodules
- ☐ Tenderness
- ☐ Other: _____

Pubococcygeus:
- ☐ Spasm
- ☐ Tenderness
- ☐ Low Tone
- ☐ Other: _____

Iliococcygeus:
- ☐ Spasm
- ☐ Tenderness
- ☐ Low tone
- ☐ Other: _____

Obturator Internus:
- ☐ Spasm
- ☐ Tenderness
- ☐ Low tone
- ☐ Other: _____

Puborectalis:
- ☐ Spasm
- ☐ Tenderness
- ☐ Low Tone
- ☐ Other: _____

Voluntary Contraction (Kegel):
- ☐ Present
- ☐ Absent
- ☐ Weak
- ☐ Strong
- ☐ Asymmetrical
- ☐ Other: _____

Anus:
- ☐ Excoriations
- ☐ Ulcerations
- ☐ Pigment changes
- ☐ Lesions
- ☐ Thickening
- ☐ Atrophy
- ☐ Masses/nodules
- ☐ Tenderness
- ☐ Loss of sensation
- ☐ Other: _____

Appendix 4

Vaginal Health Index[264]

A score of 15 or less is consistent with physical changes associated with genitourinary syndrome of menopause.

Score	Elasticity	Fluid Secretion and Consistency	pH	Epithelial Mucus	Moisture
1	None	None	>6	Petechiae noted before contact	None, mucosa inflamed
2	Poor	Scant/Thin yellow	5.6–6	Bleeds with light contact	None, mucosa not inflamed
3	Fair	Superficial/Thin white	5.1–5.5	Bleeds with scraping	Minimal
4	Good	Moderate/Thin white	4.7–5.0	Not friable, thin mucus	Moderate
5	Excellent	Normal/Flocculant white	<4–6	Not friable, normal mucosa	Normal

Appendix 5

Vulvoscopy Template

Anatomic Location	Findings						
	Excoriation	Lesion	Color Change	Mass	Ulceration	Thickening	Other
Mons Pubis							
Right Labium Magus							
Perineum							
Anus							
Left Labium Magus							
Left Infralabial Sulcus							
Posterior Commissure							
Right Infralabial Sulcus							
Anterior Commissure							

(Continued)

(Continued)

Anatomic Location	Findings						
	Excoriation	Lesion	Color Change	Mass	Ulceration	Thickening	Other
Right Labium Minus							
Posterior Fourchette							
Left Labium Minus							
Left Clitoris							
Left Vestibule							
Right Vestibule							
Right Clitoris							
Midline Vulvar Structures							

References

1. Are There More Men or Women in the World? *World Atlas* [internet]. www.world atlas.com/articles/are-there-more-men-or-women-in-the-world.html
2. Alidost F et al. Sexual Dysfunction among Women of Reproductive Age: A Systematic Review and Meta-Analysis. *International Journal of Reproductive BioMedicine*. 2021;19(5):421–432.
3. Guyer P. Kant on the Theory and Practice of Autonomy. *Social Philosophy and Policy*. 2003;20(2):70–98.
4. Egan G. *The Skilled Helper: A Systematic Approach to Effective Helping*. Monterey, CA: Brooks/Cole Pub. Co.; 1986.
5. Abbey A et al. Alcohol and Dating Risk Factors for Sexual Assault among College Women. *Psychology of Women Quarterly*. 1996;20(1):147–169.
6. Becker JV et al. Level of Postassault Sexual Functioning in Rape and Incest Victims. *Archives of Sexual Behavior*. 1986;15(1):37–49.
7. SAMHSA's Concept of Trauma and Guidance for a Trauma-Informed Approach [internet]. www.samhsa.gov/resource/dbhis/samhsas-concept-trauma-guidance-trauma-informed-approach
8. Babb C. Trauma-Informed Pelvic Exams. In: Ponce S (chair), Pelvic Pain Panel. [Symposium], Sexual Medicine Awareness Week; 2023. Keck School of Medicine, University of Southern California.
9. Medina-Martínez J et al. Health Inequities in LGBT People and Nursing Interventions to Reduce Them: A Systematic Review. *International Journal of Environmental Research and Public Health*. 2021;18(22):11801.

10. Pampati S et al. Sexual and Gender Minority Youth and Sexual Health Education: A Systematic Mapping Review of the Literature. *Journal of Adolescent Health*. 2021;68(6):1040–1052.

11. El-Hamamsy D et al. Public Understanding of Female Genital Anatomy and Pelvic Organ Prolapse (POP): A Questionnaire-Based Pilot Study. *International Urogynecology Journal*. 2022;33(2):309–318.

12. Uloko M et al. How Many Nerve Fibers Innervate the Human Glans Clitoris: A Histomorphometric Evaluation of the Dorsal Nerve of the Clitoris. *Journal of Sexual Medicine*. 2023;20(3):247–252.

13. Purves D et al. Autonomic Regulation of Sexual Function. In: *Neuroscience*. 2nd edn [internet]; 2001. www.ncbi.nlm.nih.gov/books/NBK11157/

14. Masters WH, Johnson VE. *Human Sexual Response*. Boston: Little, Brown and Company; 1966.

15. Schacter DL, Gilbert DT, Wegner DM. *Psychology*. Macmillan Higher Education; 2010.

16. By Artoria2e5 – Own Work, CC BY 3.0. https://commons.wikimedia.org/w/index.php?curid=81460023

17. Prior JC. Women's Reproductive System as Balanced Estradiol and Progesterone Actions – A Revolutionary, Paradigm-Shifting Concept in Women's Health. *Drug Discovery Today: Disease Models*. 2020;32:31–40.

18. Slob AK et al. Sexual Arousability and the Menstrual Cycle. *Psychoneuroendocrinology*. 1996;21(6):545–558.

19. Ferrante KL et al. Vaginal Estrogen for the Prevention of Recurrent Urinary Tract Infection in Postmenopausal Women: A Randomized Clinical Trial. *Female Pelvic Medicine and Reconstructive Surgery*. 2021;27(2):112–117.

20. Rosario ER et al. Brain Levels of Sex Steroid Hormones in Men and Women during Normal Aging and in Alzheimer's Disease. *Neurobiology of Aging*. 2011;32(4):604–613.

21. Anderson GL et al. Women's Health Initiative Steering Committee. Effects of Conjugated Equine Estrogen in Postmenopausal Women with Hysterectomy: The Women's Health Initiative Randomized Controlled Trial. *JAMA*. 2004; 291(14):1701–1712.

22. Writing Group for the Women's Health Initiative Investigators. Risks and Benefits of Estrogen Plus Progestin in Healthy Postmenopausal Women. JAMA. 2002;288:321–333.

23. Smoking and Breast Cancer Risk. Susan G. Komen® [internet]. www.komen.org/breast-cancer/facts-statistics/research-studies/topics/smoking-and-breast-cancer-risk/

24. O'Shaughnessy PJ et al. Alternative (Backdoor) Androgen Production and Masculinization in the Human Fetus. *PLOS Biology*. 2019;17(2):e3000002.

25. Roof RL, Hall ED. Gender Differences in Acute CNS Trauma and Stroke: Neuroprotective Effects of Estrogen and Progesterone. *Journal of Neurotrauma*. 2000;17(5):367–388.

26. Nolan BJ et al. Efficacy of Micronized Progesterone for Sleep: A Systematic Review and Meta-Analysis of Randomized Controlled Trial Data. *Journal of Clinical Endocrinology and Metabolism*. 2021;106(4):942–951.

27. Edwards M, Can AS. *Progestins*. StatPearls [internet]; 2024. www.ncbi.nlm.nih.gov/books/NBK563211/

28. Mooradian AD et al. Biological Actions of Androgens. *Endocrine Reviews*. 1987; 8(1):1–28.

29. Tobiansky DJ et al. Androgen Regulation of the Mesocorticolimbic System and Executive Function. *Frontiers in Endocrinology.* 2018;9:279.
30. van Anders SM. Testosterone and Sexual Desire in Healthy Women and Men. *Archives of Sexual Behavior.* 2012;41(6):1471–1484.
31. Moffat SD, Hampson E. A Curvilinear Relationship between Testosterone and Spatial Cognition in Humans: Possible Influence of Hand Preference. *Psychoneuroendocrinology.* 1996;21(3):323–337.
32. Cherrier MM et al. Testosterone supplementation improves spatial and verbal memory in healthy older men. *Neurology.* 2001;57(1):80–88.
33. Reed BG et al. Has Testosterone Passed the Test in Premenopausal Women with Low Libido? A Systematic Review. *International Journal of Women's Health.* 2016;8:599–607.
34. Parish SJ et al. International Society for the Study of Women's Sexual Health Clinical Practice Guideline for the Use of Systemic Testosterone for Hypoactive Sexual Desire Disorder in Women. *Journal of Sexual Medicine.* 2021;18(5):849–867.
35. Burrows LJ, Goldstein AT. The Treatment of Vestibulodynia with Topical Estradiol and Testosterone. *Sexual Medicine.* 2013;1(1):30–33.
36. Somboonporn W, Davis SR. Testosterone Effects on the Breast: Implications for Testosterone Therapy for Women. *Endocrine Reviews.* 2004;25(3):374–388.
37. Kuhl H. Pharmacology of Estrogens and Progestogens: Influence of Different Routes of Administration. *Climacteric.* 2005;8(Suppl 1):3–63.
38. Piotrowski P et al. Asp327Asn Polymorphism of Sex Hormone-Binding Globulin Gene is Associated with Systemic Lupus Erythematosus Incidence. *Molecular Biology Reports.* 2010;37(1):235–239.
39. Maggio M et al. Sex Hormone Binding Globulin Levels Across the Adult Lifespan in Women – The Role of Body Mass Index and Fasting Insulin. *Journal of Endocrinological Investigation.* 2008;31(7):597–601.
40. Selva DM, Hammond GL. Thyroid Hormones Act Indirectly to Increase Sex Hormone-Binding Globulin Production by Liver via Hepatocyte Nuclear Factor-4 alpha. *Journal of Molecular Endocrinology.* 2009;43(1):19–27.
41. Kadioglu P et al. Sexual Dysfunction in Women with Hyperprolactinemia: A Pilot Study Report. *Journal of Urology.* 2005;174(5):1921–1925.
42. Hammer F et al. No Evidence for Hepatic Conversion of Dehydroepiandrosterone (DHEA) Sulfate to DHEA: In Vivo and In Vitro Studies. *Journal of Clinical Endocrinology and Metabolism.* 2005;90(6):3600–3605.
43. Panjari M, Davis SR. DHEA Therapy for Women: Effect on Sexual Function and Wellbeing. *Human Reproduction Update.* 2007;13(3):239–248.
44. Peixoto C et al. The Effects of Dehydroepiandrosterone on Sexual Function: A Systematic Review. *Climacteric.* 2017;20(2):129–137.
45. Panjari M et al. A Randomized Trial of Oral DHEA Treatment for Sexual Function, Well-Being, and Menopausal Symptoms in Postmenopausal Women with Low Libido. *Journal of Sexual Medicine.* 2009;6(9):2579–2590.
46. Kjaergaard AD et al. Thyroid Function, Sex Hormones and Sexual Function: A Mendelian Randomization Study. *European Journal of Epidemiology.* 2021; 36(3):335–344.
47. Gabrielson AT et al. The Impact of Thyroid Disease on Sexual Dysfunction in Men and Women. *Sexual Medicine Reviews.* 2019;7(1):57–70.
48. Bates JN et al. Effect of Thyroid Hormone Derangements on Sexual Function in Men and Women. *Sexual Medicine Reviews.* 2020;8(2):217–230.

49. Krysiak R et al. Sexual Function and Depressive Symptoms in Young Women with Hypothyroidism Receiving Levothyroxine/Liothyronine Combination Therapy: A Pilot Study. *Current Medical Research and Opinion.* 2018;34(9):1579–1586.

50. Alidost F et al. Sexual Dysfunction Among Women of Reproductive Age: A Systematic Review and Meta-Analysis. *International Journal of Reproductive BioMedicine.* 2021;19(5):421–432.

51. Tripathi A et al. Biopsychosocial Model in Contemporary Psychiatry: Current Validity and Future Prospects. *Indian Journal of Psychological Medicine.* 2019;41(6):582–585.

52. Goodin BR et al. Oxytocin – A Multifunctional Analgesic for Chronic Deep Tissue Pain. *Current Pharmaceutical Design.* 2015;21(7):906–913.

53. Vowels LM et al. Uncovering the Most Important Factors for Predicting Sexual Desire Using Explainable Machine Learning. *Journal of Sexual Medicine.* 2021;18(7):1198–1216.

54. Esmat Hosseini S et al. Prevalence of Sexual Dysfunction in Women with Cancer: A Systematic Review and Meta-Analysis. *International Journal of Reproductive BioMedicine.* 2022;20(1):1–12.

55. Carter J et al. Baseline Characteristics and Concerns of Female Cancer Patients/Survivors Seeking Treatment at a Female Sexual Medicine Program. *Support Care Cancer.* 2015;23(8):2255–2265.

56. Luo F et al. Low Sexual Desire in Breast Cancer Survivors and Patients: A Review. *Sexual Medicine Reviews.* 2022;10(3):367–375.

57. Pachano Pesantez GS, Clayton AH. Treatment of Hypoactive Sexual Desire Disorder Among Women: General Considerations and Pharmacological Options. *Focus (The American Journal of Psychiatry).* 2021;19(1):39–45.

58. Segraves R, Woodard T. Female Hypoactive Sexual Desire Disorder: History and Current Status. *Journal of Sexual Medicine.* 2006;3(3):408–418.

59. West SL et al. Prevalence of Low Sexual Desire and Hypoactive Sexual Desire Disorder in a Nationally Representative Sample of US Women. *Archives of Internal Medicine.* 2008;168(13):1441–1449.

60. Pettigrew JA, Novick AM. Hypoactive Sexual Desire Disorder in Women: Physiology, Assessment, Diagnosis, and Treatment. *Journal of Midwifery & Women's Health.* 2021;66(6):740–748.

61. Pachano Pesantez GS et al. Treatment of Hypoactive Sexual Desire Disorder Among Women: General Considerations and Pharmacological Options. *Focus (The American Journal of Psychiatry).* 2021;19(1):39–45.

62. Brotto LA. The DSM diagnostic criteria for sexual aversion disorder. *Archives of Sexual Behavior.* 2010;39(2):271–277.

63. Lafortune D, et al. Prevalence and Correlates of Sexual Aversion: A Canadian Community-Based Study, *Journal of Sexual Medicine.* 2022;19(8):1269–1280.

64. Meston CM et al. *Sexual Aversion Disorder.* Austin: The Sexual Psychophysiology Laboratory, University of Texas [internet]. https://labs.la.utexas.edu/mestonlab/sexual-aversion-disorder

65. Turner D et al. The World Federation of Societies of Biological Psychiatry Guidelines on the Assessment and Pharmacological Treatment of Compulsive Sexual Behaviour Disorder. *Dialogues in Clinical Neuroscience.* 2022;24(1):10–69.

66. Fong TW. Understanding and Managing Compulsive Sexual Behaviors. *Psychiatry (Edgmont).* 2006;3(11):51–58.

67. Fuss J et al. Compulsive Sexual Behavior Disorder in Obsessive-Compulsive Disorder: Prevalence and Associated Comorbidity. *Journal of Behavioral Addictions.* 2019;8(2):242–248.

68. Kuzma JM, Black DW. Epidemiology, Prevalence, and Natural History of Compulsive Sexual Behavior. *Psychiatric Clinics of North America*. 2008;31(4):603–611.

69. Kürbitz LI, Briken P. Is Compulsive Sexual Behavior Different in Women Compared to Men? *Journal of Clinical Medicine*. 2021;10(15):3205.

70. Krueger RB, Kaplan MS. Disorders of Sexual Impulse Control in Neuropsychiatric Conditions. *Seminars in Clinical Neuropsychiatry*. 2000;5(4):266–274.

71. Seto MC et al. Assessment of the Paraphilias. *Psychiatric Clinics of North America*. 2014;37(2):149–161.

72. Kafka MP, Prentky RA. Compulsive Sexual Behavior Characteristics. *American Journal of Psychiatry*. 1997;154(11):1632.

73. Bergner RM. Sexual Compulsion as Attempted Recovery from Degradation: Theory and Therapy. *Journal of Sex & Marital Therapy*. 2002;28(5):373–387.

74. Landgren V et al. Pharmacological Treatment for Pedophilic Disorder and Compulsive Sexual Behavior Disorder: A Review. *Drugs*. 2022;82(6):663–681.

75. Weiss P, Brody S. Female Sexual Arousal Disorder with and without a Distress Criterion: Prevalence and Correlates in a Representative Czech Sample. *Journal of Sexual Medicine*. 2009;6(12):3385–3394.

76. Meston CM, Stanton AM. Understanding Sexual Arousal and Subjective-Genital Arousal Desynchrony in Women. *Nature Reviews Urology*. 2019;16(2):107–120.

77. Holub AM. Plethysmography. Encyclopedia of Personality and Individual Differences. In: *Encyclopedia of Personality and Individual Differences* [internet]; 2017. https://doi.org/10.1007/978-3-319-28099-8_795-1

78. Lovie K, Marashi A. Coital Positions and Clitoral Blood Flow: A Biomechanical and Sonographic Analysis. *Sexologies*. 2022;31(4):423–429.

79. Meldrum DR et al. The Link between Erectile and Cardiovascular Health: The Canary in the Coal Mine. *American Journal of Cardiology*. 2011;108(4):599–606.

80. Park K et al. Vasculogenic Female Sexual Dysfunction: The Hemodynamic Basis for Vaginal Engorgement Insufficiency and Clitoral Erectile Insufficiency. *International Journal of Impotence Research*. 1997;9(1):27–37 [published correction appears in *International Journal of Impotence Research*. 1998;10(1):67].

81. Rupp HA, Wallen K. Sex Differences in Response to Visual Sexual Stimuli: A Review. *Archives of Sexual Behavior*. 2008;37(2):206–218.

82. Basson R. The Female Sexual Response: A Different Model. *Journal of Sex & Marital Therapy*. 2000;26(1):51–65.

83. Bancroft J et al. Distress about Sex: A National Survey of Women in Heterosexual Relationships. *Archives of Sexual Behavior*. 2003;32(3):193–208.

84. Labrie F. DHEA, Important Source of Sex Steroids in Men and Even More in Women. *Progress in Brain Research*. 2010;182:97–148.

85. Chivers ML. A Brief Review and Discussion of Sex Differences in the Specificity of Sexual Arousal. *Sexual and Relationship Therapy*. 2005;20(4):377–390.

86. Tan-Kim J et al. Efficacy of Vaginal Estrogen for Recurrent Urinary Tract Infection Prevention in Hypoestrogenic Women. *American Journal of Obstetrics and Gynecology*. 2023;229(2):143.e1–143.e9.

87. Goldstein I et al. International Society for the Study of Women's Sexual Health (ISSWSH) Review of Epidemiology and Pathophysiology, and a Consensus Nomenclature and Process of Care for the Management of Persistent Genital Arousal Disorder/Genito-Pelvic Dysesthesia (PGAD/GPD). *Journal of Sexual Medicine*. 2021;18(4):665–697.

88. Jackowich RA et al. Healthcare Experiences of Individuals with Persistent Genital Arousal Disorder/Genito-Pelvic Dysesthesia. *Sexual Medicine*. 2021;9(3):100335.

89. Leiblum S et al. Persistent Sexual Arousal Syndrome: A Descriptive Study. *Journal of Sexual Medicine*. 2005;2(3):331–337.

90. Jackowich RA et al. A Comparison of Medical Comorbidities, Psychosocial, and Sexual Well-Being in an Online Cross-Sectional Sample of Women Experiencing Persistent Genital Arousal Symptoms and a Control Group. *Journal of Sexual Medicine*. 2020;17(1):69–82.

91. Franklin B. *The Works of Benjamin Franklin . . . Published with Notes and a Life of the Author by Jared Sparks*; 1840.

92. Cordell WH et al. The High Prevalence of Pain in Emergency Medical Care. *American Journal of Emergency Medicine*. 2002;20(3):165–169.

93. Weijmar Schultz W et al. Women's Sexual Pain and Its Management. *Journal of Sexual Medicine*. 2005;2(3):301–316.

94. Soni KK et al. Neurons for Ejaculation and Factors Affecting Ejaculation. *Biology*. 2022;11(5):686.

95. Garland EL. Pain Processing in the Human Nervous System: A Selective Review of Nociceptive and Biobehavioral Pathways. *Primary Care*. 2012;39(3):561–571.

96. Rathus SA et al. *Human Sexuality in a World of Diversity*. 6th edn. Pearson; 2020.

97. Haefner HK. Report of the International Society for the Study of Vulvovaginal Disease Terminology and Classification of Vulvodynia. *Journal of Lower Genital Tract Disease*. 2007;11(1):48–49.

98. Sadownik LA. Etiology, Diagnosis, and Clinical Management of Vulvodynia. *International Journal of Women's Health*. 2014;6:437–449.

99. Chadha S et al. Histopathologic Features of Vulvar Vestibulitis. *International Journal of Gynecological Pathology*. 1998;17(1):7–11.

100. Hampson JP et al. Augmented Central Pain Processing in Vulvodynia. *Journal of Pain*. 2013;14(6):579–589.

101. Bergeron S et al. A Randomized Comparison of Group Cognitive–Behavioral Therapy, Surface Electromyographic Biofeedback, and Vestibulectomy in the Treatment of Dyspareunia Resulting from Vulvar Vestibulitis. *Pain*. 2001;91(3):297–306.

102. Leo RJ, Dewani S. A Systematic Review of the Utility of Antidepressant Pharmacotherapy in the Treatment of Vulvodynia Pain. *Journal of Sexual Medicine*. 2013;10(10):2497–2505.

103. Leo RJ. A Systematic Review of the Utility of Anticonvulsant Pharmacotherapy in the Treatment of Vulvodynia Pain. *Journal of Sexual Medicine*. 2013;10(8):2000–2008.

104. Andrews JC. Vulvodynia Interventions – Systematic Review and Evidence Grading. *Obstetrical & Gynecological Survey*. 2011;66(5):299–315.

105. American Psychiatric Association. *DSM-5 TM Guidebook the Essential Companion to the Diagnostic and Statistical Manual of Mental Disorders*. 5th ed. Washington, DC, American Psychiatric Publishing; 2013.

106. Pacik PT et al. Case Series: Redefining Severe Grade 5 Vaginismus. *Sexual Medicine*. 2019;7(4):489–497.

107. eissing ED et al. "Throwing the Baby Out with the Bathwater": The Demise of Vaginismus in Favor of Genito-Pelvic Pain/Penetration Disorder. *Archives of Sexual Behavior*. 2014;43(7):1209–1213.

108. Spoelstra SK. *The Genito-Pelvic Pain/Penetration Disorder Paradigm and Beyond: Theoretical and Empirical Perspectives*. University of Groningen Research Portal [internet]; 2017. https://hdl.handle.net/11370/831b3f64-9a58-42b3-82d3-9c949e171958

109. McEvoy M et al. Understanding Vaginismus: A Biopsychosocial Perspective. *Sexual and Relationship Therapy*. 2023;39(3):680–701.

110. Babb C. Vaginismus. *Prosayla.com* [internet]; 2019. www.prosayla.com/articles/vaginismus

111. Pacik PT et al. Case Series: Redefining Severe Grade 5 Vaginismus. *Sexual Medicine.* 2019;7(4):489–497.

112. Brin MF, Vapnek JM. Treatment of Vaginismus with Botulinum Toxin Injections. *Lancet.* 1997;349(9047):252–253 [published correction appears in *Lancet.* 1997; 349(9052):656].

113. Pacik PT. Understanding and Treating Vaginismus: A Multimodal Approach. *International Urogynecology Journal.* 2014;25(12):1613–1620.

114. Faubion SS et al. Recognition and Management of Nonrelaxing Pelvic Floor Dysfunction. *Mayo Clinic Proceedings.* 2012;87(2):187–193.

115. Grimes WR, Stratton M. *Pelvic Floor Dysfunction.* StatPearls [internet]; 2023. www.ncbi.nlm.nih.gov/books/NBK559246/

116. Good MM, Solomon ER. Pelvic Floor Disorders. *Obstetrics and Gynecology Clinics of North America.* 2019;46(3):527–540.

117. Faubion SS et al. Recognition and Management of Nonrelaxing Pelvic Floor Dysfunction. *Mayo Clinic Proceedings.* 2012;87(2):187–193.

118. Pomian A et al. Obesity and Pelvic Floor Disorders: A Review of the Literature. *Medical Science Monitor.* 2016;22:1880–1886.

119. Silantyeva E et al. A Comparative Study on the Effects of High-Intensity Focused Electromagnetic Technology and Electrostimulation for the Treatment of Pelvic Floor Muscles and Urinary Incontinence in Parous Women: Analysis of Posttreatment Data. *Female Pelvic Medicine and Reconstructive Surgery.* 2021;27(4):269–273.

120. Desrosiers L, Knoepp LR. Botulinum Toxin A: A Review of Potential Uses in Treatment of Female Urogenital and Pelvic Floor Disorders. *Ochsner Journal.* 2020;20(4):400–409.

121. Purwar B, Khullar V. Use of Botulinum Toxin for Chronic Pelvic Pain. *Womens Health.* 2016;12(3):293–296.

122. Carter A et al. "Fulfilling His Needs, Not Mine": Reasons for Not Talking about Painful Sex and Associations with Lack of Pleasure in a Nationally Representative Sample of Women in the United States. *Journal of Sexual Medicine.* 2019;16(12):1953–1965.

123. Thompson CM et al. Women's Experiences of Health-Related Communicative Disenfranchisement. *Health Communication.* 2023;38(14):3135–3146.

124. Ovid. *Ovid's Metamorphoses: Translated by Eminent Persons.* 4 Volumes. Sir Samuel Garth; 1794.

125. Matthews G, Everest K. *The Poems of Shelley.* Volume 1. Routledge; 2014.

126. Mintz LB. *Becoming Cliterate: Why Orgasm Equality Matters – And How to Get It.* Harperone; 2018.

127. Masters WH, Johnson VE, *Human Sexual Response.* Little Brown; 1966.

128. van Netten JJ et al. 8–13 Hz Fluctuations in Rectal Pressure Are an Objective Marker of Clitorally Induced Orgasm in Women. *Archives of Sexual Behavior.* 2008;37(2):279–285.

129. Levin RJ, Wagner G. Orgasm in Women in the Laboratory – Quantitative Studies on Duration, Intensity, Latency, and Vaginal Blood Flow. *Archives of Sexual Behavior.* 1985;14(5):439–449.

130. Miller G. *The Mating Mind: How Sexual Choice Shaped the Evolution of Human Nature.* Vintage; 2001.

131. Baker RR, Bellis MA. Human Sperm Competition: Ejaculate Manipulation by Females and a Function for the Female Orgasm. *Animal Behaviour.* 1993;46(5):887–909.

132. Wise NJ et al. Brain Activity Unique to Orgasm in Women: An fMRI Analysis. *Journal of Sexual Medicine.* 2017;14(11):1380–1391.

133. Kruger D, Hughes SM. Variation in Reproductive Strategies Influences Post-Coital Experiences with Partners. *Journal of Social, Evolutionary, and Cultural Psychology.* 2010;4:254–264.

134. Humphries AK, Cioe J. Reconsidering the Refractory Period: An Exploratory Study of Women's Post-Orgasmic Experiences. *Canadian Journal of Human Sexuality.* 2009;18:127.

135. Opperman E et al. "It Feels so Good It Almost Hurts": Young Adults' Experiences of Orgasm and Sexual Pleasure. *Journal of Sex Research.* 2014;51(5):503–515.

136. Séguin LJ et al. Consuming Ecstasy: Representations of Male and Female Orgasm in Mainstream Pornography. *Journal of Sex Research.* 2018;55(3):348–356.

137. Kinsey AC et al. *Sexual Behavior in the Human Female.* Saunders; 1953.

138. Döring N, Mohseni R. Der Gender Orgasm Gap. Ein kritischer Forschungsüberblick zu Geschlechterdifferenzen in der Orgasmus-Häufigkeit beim Heterosex. *Zeitschrift für Sexualforschung.* 2022;35(2):73–87.

139. Pfaus JG et al. The Whole versus the Sum of Some of the Parts: Toward Resolving the Apparent Controversy of Clitoral versus Vaginal Orgasms. *Socioaffective Neuroscience & Psychology.* 2016;6:32578.

140. Moore L, Clarke A. Clitoral Conventions and Transgressions: Graphic Representations in Anatomy Texts, c1900–1991. *Feminist Studies.* 1995;21(2):255.

141. Scully D, Bart P. A Funny Thing Happened on the Way to the Orifice: Women in Gynecology Textbooks. *AJS.* 1973;78(4):1045–1050.

142. Herbenick D et al. Women's Experiences with Genital Touching, Sexual Pleasure, and Orgasm: Results From a U.S. Probability Sample of Women Ages 18 to 94. *Journal of Sex & Marital Therapy.* 2018;44(2):201–212.

143. Hensel DJ et al. Women's Techniques for Making Vaginal Penetration More Pleasurable: Results from a Nationally Representative Study of Adult Women in the United States. *PLoS One.* 2021;16(4):e0249242.

144. Meston CM et al. Disorders of Orgasm in Women. *Journal of Sexual Medicine.* 2004;1(1):66–68.

145. McCabe MP et al. Incidence and Prevalence of Sexual Dysfunction in Women and Men: A Consensus Statement from the Fourth International Consultation on Sexual Medicine 2015. *Journal of Sexual Medicine.* 2016;13(2):144–152.

146. Meston C, Stanton A. *Female Orgasmic Disorder.* Austin: The Sexual Psychophysiology Laboratory, University of Texas [internet]. https://labs.la.utexas.edu/mestonlab/female-orgasmic-disorder/

147. Basson R, Schultz WW. Sexual Sequelae of General Medical Disorders. *Lancet.* 2007;369(9559):409–424.

148. Stimmel GL, Gutierrez MA. Sexual Dysfunction and Psychotropic Medications. *CNS Spectrums.* 2006;11(Suppl 9):24–30.

149. Ingram CF et al. Testosterone Therapy and Other Treatment Modalities for Female Sexual Dysfunction. *Current Opinion in Urology.* 2020;30(3):309–316.

150. Meston CM et al. Women's Orgasm. *Annual Review of Sex Research.* 2004;15:173–257.

151. Goodman MP et al. Evaluation of Body Image and Sexual Satisfaction in Women Undergoing Female Genital Plastic/Cosmetic Surgery. *Aesthetic Surgery Journal.* 2016;36(9):1048–1057.

152. Binik YM, Hall KSK. *Principles and Practice of Sex Therapy.* Guilford Press; 2020.

153. Behnia B et al. Differential Effects of Intranasal Oxytocin on Sexual Experiences and Partner Interactions in Couples. *Hormones and Behavior*. 2014;65(3):308–318.

154. Sukgen G et al. Platelet-Rich Plasma Administration to the Lower Anterior Vaginal Wall to Improve Female Sexuality Satisfaction. *Turkish Journal of Obstetrics and Gynecology*. 2019;16(4):228–234.

155. Lynn BK et al. The Relationship between Marijuana Use Prior to Sex and Sexual Function in Women. *Sexual Medicine*. 2019;7(2):192–197.

156. Zimmerman LL et al. Transcutaneous Electrical Nerve Stimulation to Improve Female Sexual Dysfunction Symptoms: A Pilot Study. *Neuromodulation*. 2018; 21(7):707–713.

157. Chaukimath SP, Patil PS. Orgasm-Induced Seizures: A Rare Phenomenon. *Annals of Medical and Health Science Research*. 2015;5(6):483–484. https://doi.org/10.4103/2141-9248.177993

158. Reynolds MR, Willie JT, Zipfel GJ, Dacey RG. Sexual Intercourse and Cerebral Aneurysmal Rupture: Potential Mechanisms and Precipitants. *Journal of Neurosurgery*. 2011;114(4):969–977. https://doi.org/10.3171/2010.4.JNS09975

159. Perelman M. *Orgasmic Anhedonia/PDOD: Causes*. www.sexualmed.org [Published April 15, 2013. Accessed October 15, 2024. www.sexualmed.org/index.cfm/sexual-health-issues/for-men/anhedoniapdod/treatment/]

160. Schaumburg H et al. Sensory Neuropathy from Pyridoxine Abuse. A New Megavitamin Syndrome. *New England Journal of Medicine*. 1983;309(8):445–448.

161. Herbenick D et al. Women's Sexual Satisfaction, Communication, and Reasons for (No Longer) Faking Orgasm: Findings from a U.S. Probability Sample. *Archives of Sexual Behavior*. 2019;48(8):2461–2472.

162. Jonason PK. Reasons to Pretend to Orgasm and the Mating Psychology of Those Who Endorse Them. *Personality and Individual Differences*. 2019;143:90–94.

163. Aishworiya R et al. An Update on Psychopharmacological Treatment of Autism Spectrum Disorder. *Neurotherapeutics*. 2022;19(1):248–262.

164. Connor H. Medieval Uroscopy and Its Representation on Misericords–Part 1: Uroscopy. *Journal of Clinical Medicine*. 2001;1(6):507–509.

165. Armstrong JA. Urinalysis in Western Culture: A Brief History. *Kidney International*. 2007;71(5):384–387.

166. Horowitz GL. Reference Intervals: Practical Aspects. *EJIFCC*. 2008;19(2):95–105.

167. Find a Test. *Labcorp* [internet]. www.labcorp.com/test-menu/search

168. Reginster JY et al. Minimal Levels of Serum Estradiol Prevent Postmenopausal Bone Loss. *Calcified Tissue International*. 1992;51(5):340–343.

169. Azadzoi KM, Siroky MB. Neurologic Factors in Female Sexual Function and Dysfunction. *Korean Journal of Urology*. 2010;51(7):443–449.

170. Mechelmans DJ et al. The Successful Measurement of Clitoral Pulse Amplitude Using a New Clitoral Photoplethysmograph: A Pilot Study. *Journal of Sexual Medicine*. 2020;17(6):1118–1125.

171. Yoon I, Gupta N. *Pelvic Prolapse Imaging*. StatPearls [internet]; 2023. www.ncbi.nlm.nih.gov/books/NBK551513/

172. El Sayed RF et al. Magnetic Resonance Imaging of Pelvic Floor Dysfunction – Joint Recommendations of the ESUR and ESGAR Pelvic Floor Working Group. *European Radiology*. 2017;27(5):2067–2085.

173. Ruesink GB, Georgiadis JR. Brain Imaging of Human Sexual Response: Recent Developments and Future Directions. *Current Sexual Health Reports*. 2017;9(4):183–191.

174. Calabrò RS. Sexual Dysfunction in Neurological Disorders: Do We See Just the Tip of the Iceberg? *Acta Biomedica*. 2018;89(2):274–275.

175. Schultz WW et al. Magnetic Resonance Imaging of Male and Female Genitals during Coitus and Female Sexual Arousal. *BMJ*. 1999;319(7225):1596–1600.

176. Goldstein I et al. International Society for the Study of Women's Sexual Health (ISSWSH) Review of Epidemiology and Pathophysiology, and a Consensus Nomenclature and Process of Care for the Management of Persistent Genital Arousal Disorder/Genito-Pelvic Dysesthesia (PGAD/GPD). *Journal of Sexual Medicine*. 2021;18(4):665–697.

177. Gerritsen J et al. The Clitoral Photoplethysmograph: A New Way of Assessing Genital Arousal in Women. *Journal of Sexual Medicine*. 2009;6(6):1678–1687.

178. Laan E et al. Assessment of Female Sexual Arousal: Response Specificity and Construct Validity. *Psychophysiology*. 1995;32(5):476–485.

179. Ghanavatian S et al. *Pudendal Nerve Block*. StatPearls [internet]; 2023. www.ncbi.nlm.nih.gov/books/NBK551518/

180. Carrico DJ, Peters KM. Vaginal Diazepam Use with Urogenital Pain/Pelvic Floor Dysfunction: Serum Diazepam Levels and Efficacy Data. *Urologic Nursing*. 2011;31(5):279–299.

181. Larish AM et al. Vaginal Diazepam for Nonrelaxing Pelvic Floor Dysfunction: The Pharmacokinetic Profile. *Journal of Sexual Medicine*. 2019;16(6):763–766.

182. Bao C et al. Provoked Vestibulodynia in Women with Pelvic Pain. *Sexual Medicine*. 2019;7(2):227–234.

183. Hardy JD. *Pain Sensations and Reactions*. Williams & Wilkins; 1952.

184. Cohen K. *The Way of Qigong = [Ch'i Kung Chi Tao]: The Art and Science of Chinese Energy Healing*. Ballantine Books; 1997.

185. Goldštajn MŠ et al. Effects of Transdermal versus Oral Hormone Replacement Therapy in Postmenopause: A Systematic Review. *Archives of Gynecology and Obstetrics*. 2023;307(6):1727–1745.

186. Davis SR et al. Effects of Estradiol with and without Testosterone on Body Composition and Relationships with Lipids in Postmenopausal Women. *Menopause*. 2000;7(6):395–401.

187. Obata H. Analgesic Mechanisms of Antidepressants for Neuropathic Pain. *International Journal of Molecular Sciences*. 2017;18(11):2483.

188. Loflin BJ et al. Vulvodynia: A Review of the Literature. *Journal of Pharmacy Technology*. 2019;35(1):11–24.

189. Hameroff SR et al. Doxepin's Effects on Chronic Pain and Depression: A Controlled Study. *Journal of Clinical Psychiatry*. 1984;45(3 Pt 2):47–53.

190. Kerr GW et al. Tricyclic Antidepressant Overdose: A Review. *Emergency Medicine Journal*. 2001;18(4):236–241.

191. Razali NA et al. The Role of Bupropion in the Treatment of Women with Sexual Desire Disorder: A Systematic Review and Meta-Analysis. *Current Neuropharmacology*. 2022;20(10):1941–1955.

192. Romanello JP et al. Clitoral Adhesions: A Review of the Literature. *Sexual Medicine Reviews*. 2023;11(3):196–201.

193. Aboud C et al. Surgical Treatment of Clitoral Phimosis. *Journal of Gynecology Obstetrics and Human Reproduction*. 2021;50(6):101919.

194. Halperin R et al. The Major Histopathologic Characteristics in the Vulvar Vestibulitis Syndrome. *Gynecologic and Obstetric Investigation*. 2005;59(2):75–79.

195. Goetsch MF. Incidence of Bartholin's Duct Occlusion after Superficial Localized Vestibulectomy. *American Journal of Obstetrics and Gynecology.* 2009;200(6):688. e1–688.e6886.

196. Parish SJ et al. International Society for the Study of Women's Sexual Health Clinical Practice Guideline for the Use of Systemic Testosterone for Hypoactive Sexual Desire Disorder in Women. *Journal of Sexual Medicine.* 2021;18(5):849–867.

197. Quirk FH et al. Development of a Sexual Function Questionnaire for Clinical Trials of Female Sexual Dysfunction. *Journal of Women's Health & Gender-Based Medicine.* 2002;11(3):277–289.

198. Symonds T et al. Sexual Function Questionnaire: Further Refinement and Validation. *Journal of Sexual Medicine.* 2012;9(10):2609–2616.

199. Rosen R et al. The Female Sexual Function Index (FSFI): A Multidimensional Self-Report Instrument for the Assessment of Female Sexual Function. *Journal of Sex & Marital Therapy.* 2000;26(2):191–208.

200. Clayton AH et al. Validation of the Decreased Sexual Desire Screener (DSDS): A Brief Diagnostic Instrument for Generalized Acquired Female Hypoactive Sexual Desire Disorder (HSDD). *Journal of Sexual Medicine.* 2009;6(3):730–738.

201. Spector IP et al. The Sexual Desire Inventory: Development, Factor Structure, and Evidence of Reliability. *Journal of Sex & Marital Therapy.* 1996;22(3):175–190.

202. Toledano R, Pfaus J. The Sexual Arousal and Desire Inventory (SADI): A Multidimensional Scale to Assess Subjective Sexual Arousal and Desire. *Journal of Sexual Medicine.* 2006;3(5):853–877.

203. Mah K, Binik YM. Do All Orgasms Feel Alike? Evaluating a Two-Dimensional Model of the Orgasm Experience across Gender and Sexual Context. *Journal of Sex Research.* 2002;39(2):104–113.

204. Mah K, Binik YM. The Nature of Human Orgasm: A Critical Review of Major Trends. *Clinical Psychology Review.* 2001;21(6):823–856.

205. McIntyre-Smith A, Fisher W. Female Partner's Communication during Sexual Scale Activity. In: Fisher TD et al. (eds), *Handbook of Sexuality – Related Measures.* 3rd edn. Routledge; 2010:134–136.

206. Hudson WW et al. A Short-Form Scale to Measure Sexual Discord in Dyadic Relationships. *Journal of Sex Research.* 1981;17(2):157–174.

207. Molaeinezhad M et al. Development and Validation of the Multidimensional Vaginal Penetration Disorder Questionnaire (MVPDQ) for Assessment of Lifelong Vaginismus in a Sample of Iranian Women. *Journal of Research in Medical Sciences.* 2014;19(4):336–348.

208. Grover S, Shouan A. Assessment Scales for Sexual Disorders – A Review. *Journal of Psychosexual Health.* 2020;2(2):263183182091958.

209. Connolly B. What Did Ancient Babylonians Eat? A Yale-Harvard Team Tested Their Recipes. *Yale News* [internet]; 2018. https://news.yale.edu/2018/06/14/what-did-ancient-babylonians-eat-yale-harvard-team-tested-their-recipes

210. Bauer SR et al. Association of Diet with Erectile Dysfunction among Men in the Health Professionals Follow-Up Study. *JAMA Network Open.* 2020;3(11):e2021701.

211. Scavello I et al. Cardiometabolic Risk is Unraveled by Color Doppler Ultrasound of the Clitoral and Uterine Arteries in Women Consulting for Sexual Symptoms. *Scientific Reports.* 2021;11(1):18899.

212. Buettner D, Skemp S. Blue Zones: Lessons from the World's Longest Lived. *American Journal of Lifestyle Medicine.* 2016;10(5):318–321.

213. Castro AI et al. Effect of a Very Low-Calorie Ketogenic Diet on Food and Alcohol Cravings, Physical and Sexual Activity, Sleep Disturbances, and Quality of Life in Obese Patients. *Nutrients*. 2018;10(10):1348.

214. Esposito K et al. Mediterranean Diet Improves Sexual Function in Women with the Metabolic Syndrome. *International Journal of Impotence Research*. 2007; 19(5):486–491.

215. Mishra S et al. Dietary Supplement Use among Adults: United States, 2017–2018. *NCHS Data Brief*. 2021;399:1–8.

216. Jenkins L et al. AUA2022: REFLECTIONS: The Safety and Efficacy of Sexual Supplements. *AUANews*; 2022. https://auanews.net/issues/articles/2022/august-2022/aua2022-reflections-the-safety-and-efficacy-of-sexual-supplements

217. Cieri-Hutcherson NE et al. Systematic Review of L-Arginine for the Treatment of Hypoactive Sexual Desire Disorder and Related Conditions in Women. *Pharmacy*. 2021;9(2):71.

218. Chiang VS, Park JH. Glutamate in Male and Female Sexual Behavior: Receptors, Transporters, and Steroid Independence. *Frontiers in Behavioral Neuroscience*. 2020;14:589882.

219. Shin BC et al. Maca (L. meyenii) for Improving Sexual Function: A Systematic Review. *BMC Complementary and Alternative Medicine*. 2010;10:44.

220. Estrada-Reyes R et al. *Turnera diffusa* Wild (Turneraceae) Recovers Sexual Behavior in Sexually Exhausted Males. *Journal of Ethnopharmacology*. 2009;123(3): 423–429.

221. Ito TY et al. A Double-Blind Placebo-Controlled Study of ArginMax, a Nutritional Supplement for Enhancement of Female Sexual Function. *Journal of Sex & Marital Therapy*. 2001;27(5):541–549.

222. Martimbianco ALC et al. *Tribulus terrestris* for Female Sexual Dysfunction: A Systematic Review. *Tribulus terrestris* Para disfunção Sexual Feminina: Uma Revisão Sistemática. *Revista Brasileira de Ginecologia e Obstetrícia*. 2020; 42(7):427–435.

223. Gama CR et al. Clinical Assessment of *Tribulus terrestris* Extract in the Treatment of Female Sexual Dysfunction. *Clinical Medicine Insights: Women's Health*. 2014;7:45–50.

224. Oh KJ et al. Effects of Korean Red Ginseng on Sexual Arousal in Menopausal Women: Placebo-Controlled, Double-Blind Crossover Clinical Study. *Journal of Sexual Medicine*. 2010;7(4 Pt 1):1469–1477.

225. Rao A et al. Influence of a Specialized *Trigonella foenum* Graecum Seed Extract (Libifem), on Testosterone, Estradiol and Sexual Function in Healthy Menstruating Women, a Randomised Placebo Controlled Study. *Phytotherapy Research*. 2015;29(8):1123–1130.

226. Dongre S et al. Efficacy and Safety of Ashwagandha (*Withania somnifera*) Root Extract in Improving Sexual Function in Women: A Pilot Study. *BioMed Research International*. 2015;2015:284154.

227. Ajgaonkar A et al. Efficacy and Safety of Ashwagandha (*Withania somnifera*) Root Extract for Improvement of Sexual Health in Healthy Women: A Prospective, Randomized, Placebo-Controlled Study. *Cureus*. 2022;14(10):e30787.

228. Meston CM et al. Short- and Long-Term Effects of Ginkgo Biloba Extract on Sexual Dysfunction in Women. *Archives of Sexual Behavior*. 2008;37(4):530–547.

229. Cui T et al. A Urologist's Guide to Ingredients Found in Top-Selling Nutraceuticals for Men's Sexual Health. *Journal of Sexual Medicine*. 2015;12(11):2105–2117.

230. Bechara N et al. A Systematic Review on the Role of Vitamin C in Tissue Healing. *Antioxidants.* 2022;11(8):1605.
231. Chu C et al. Relationship between Vitamin D and Hormones Important for Human Fertility in Reproductive-Aged Women. *Frontiers in Endocrinology.* 2021;12:666687.
232. Te L et al. Correlation between Serum Zinc and Testosterone: A Systematic Review. *Journal of Trace Elements in Medicine and Biology.* 2023;76:127124.
233. Mazaheri Nia L et al. Effect of Zinc on Testosterone Levels and Sexual Function of Postmenopausal Women: A Randomized Controlled Trial. *Journal of Sex & Marital Therapy.* 2021;47(8):804–813.
234. Seelig MS. Interrelationship of Magnesium and Estrogen in Cardiovascular and Bone Disorders, Eclampsia, Migraine and Premenstrual Syndrome. *Journal of the American College of Nutrition.* 1993;12(4):442–458.
235. Nikzad Z et al. The Relationship between Iron Deficiency Anemia and Sexual Function and Satisfaction among Reproductive-Aged Iranian Women. *PLoS One.* 2018;13(12):e0208485.
236. Palmeri ST et al. Heart Rate and Blood Pressure Response in Adult Men and Women during Exercise and Sexual Activity. *American Journal of Cardiology.* 2007;100(12):1795–1801.
237. Carcelén-Fraile MDC et al. Effects of Physical Exercise on Sexual Function and Quality of Sexual Life Related to Menopausal Symptoms in Peri- and Postmenopausal Women: A Systematic Review. *International Journal of Environmental Research and Public Health.* 2020;17(8):2680.
238. Syed AH et al. Association of Weight Loss with Improved Sexual Function in Females. *Cureus.* 2021;13(8):c16849.
239. Stanton AM et al. The Effects of Exercise on Sexual Function in Women. *Sexual Medicine Reviews.* 2018;6(4):548–557.
240. Medic G et al. Short- and Long-Term Health Consequences of Sleep Disruption. *Nature and Science of Sleep.* 2017;9:151–161.
241. Kalmbach DA et al. The Impact of Sleep on Female Sexual Response and Behavior: A Pilot Study. *Journal of Sexual Medicine.* 2015;12(5):1221–1232.
242. Buckley TM, Schatzberg AF. On the Interactions of the Hypothalamic-Pituitary-Adrenal (HPA) Axis and Sleep: Normal HPA Axis Activity and Circadian Rhythm, Exemplary Sleep Disorders. *Journal of Clinical Endocrinology and Metabolism.* 2005;90(5):3106–3114.
243. Lateef OM, Akintubosun MO. Sleep and Reproductive Health. *Journal of Circadian Rhythms.* 2020;18:1.
244. Whale K, Gooberman-Hill R. The Importance of Sleep for People with Chronic Pain: Current Insights and Evidence. *JBMR Plus.* 2022;6(7):e10658.
245. Breton A et al. Enhancing the Sexual Function of Women Living with Chronic Pain: A Cognitive-Behavioural Treatment Group. *Pain Research and Management.* 2008;13(3):219–224.
246. Suni E, Singh A. *20 Tips for How to Sleep Better.* Sleep Foundation [internet]; 2023. www.sleepfoundation.org/sleep-hygiene/healthy-sleep-tips
247. Roberts BL, Karatsoreos IN. Brain-Body Responses to Chronic Stress: A Brief Review. *Faculty Reviews.* 2021;10:83.
248. Hamilton LD, Meston CM. Chronic Stress and Sexual Function in Women. *Journal of Sexual Medicine.* 2013;10(10):2443–2454.
249. Arcos-Romero AI, Calvillo C. Sexual Health and Psychological Well-Being of Women: A Systematic Review. *Healthcare.* 2023;11(23):3025.

250. Wagnild GM, Young HM. Development and Psychometric Evaluation of the Resilience Scale. *Journal of Nursing Measurement*. 1993;1(2):165–178.

251. Sood R et al. Association of Resilience with Female Sexual Dysfunction. *Maturitas*. 2024;183:107939.

252. van Woudenberg C et al. The Impact of Intensive Trauma-Focused Treatment on Sexual Functioning in Individuals with PTSD. *Frontiers in Psychology*. 2023; 14:1191916.

253. O'Callaghan E et al. Navigating Sex and Sexuality after Sexual Assault: A Qualitative Study of Survivors and Informal Support Providers. *Journal of Sex Research*. 2019;56(8):1045–1057.

254. Bird ER et al. Relationship between Posttraumatic Stress Disorder and Sexual Difficulties: A Systematic Review of Veterans and Military Personnel. *Journal of Sexual Medicine*. 2021;18(8):1398–1426.

255. Cichowski SB et al. Sexual Abuse History and Pelvic Floor Disorders in Women. *Southern Medical Journal*. 2013;106(12):675–678.

256. Beck JJ et al. Multiple Pelvic Floor Complaints Are Correlated with Sexual Abuse History. *Journal of Sexual Medicine*. 2009;6(1):193–198.

257. Pergament D. Exactly How Much Appearance Matters, According to Our National Judgment Survey. *Allure* [internet]; 2016. www.allure.com/story/national-judgement-survey-statistics

258. McCabe MP et al. Where Is All the Pressure Coming From? Messages from Mothers and Teachers about Preschool Children's Appearance, Diet and Exercise. *European Eating Disorders Review*. 2007;15(3):221–230.

259. Tort-Nasarre G et al. The Meaning and Factors That Influence the Concept of Body Image: Systematic Review and Meta-Ethnography from the Perspectives of Adolescents. *International Journal of Environmental Research and Public Health*. 2021;18(3):1140.

260. Woertman L, van den Brink F. Body Image and Female Sexual Functioning and Behavior: A Review. *Journal of Sex Research*. 2012;49(2–3):184–211.

261. Quinn-Nilas C et al. The Relationship Between Body Image and Domains of Sexual Functioning among Heterosexual, Emerging Adult Women. *Sexual Medicine*. 2016;4(3):e182–e189.

262. Horvath Z et al. Body Image, Orgasmic Response, and Sexual Relationship Satisfaction: Understanding Relationships and Establishing Typologies Based on Body Image Satisfaction. *Sexual Medicine*. 2020;8(4):740–751.

263. Maslow A. *Theory of Human Motivation*. Volume 50. Wilder Publications; 1943: 370–396.

264. Hess R, et al. Vaginal Maturation Index Self-Sample Collection in Mid-Life Women: Acceptability and Correlation with Physician-Collected Samples. *Menopause*. 2008;15(4 Pt 1):726–729.

Index

Note: Page numbers in *italics* indicate a figure and page numbers in **bold** indicate a table on the corresponding page.

For Product Safety Concerns and Information please contact our EU
representative GPSR@taylorandfrancis.com
Taylor & Francis Verlag GmbH, Kaufingerstraße 24, 80331 München, Germany